Fabulous
IN FLATS

How I've Learned to
Thrive While Living with an
Autoimmune Illness

KELLI GASTIS

FABULOUS IN FLATS

How I've Learned to Thrive While
Living with an Autoimmune Illness

ISBN PRINT: 978-1-990352-88-1

Art Direction including Book Cover,
Typesetting and Layout Design
Copyright © 2023, LeadHer Publishing
Graphic Design - Christina Williams
Editing - Donna Zuniga, Megan Jackson
Photography - Leah Smith

To find out more about Kelli Gastis, visit www.kelligastis.com
To find out more about the publisher, visit www.leadherpublishing.com

Disclaimer

The content presented in this book, Fabulous in Flats, is provided as a resource only. It is not meant to replace professional medical advice, diagnosis, or treatment. Any attempt to diagnose and/or treat a medical condition should be done under the direction of a healthcare provider or physician. For any medical conditions, each individual is recommended to consult with a healthcare provider before using any information, idea, or methods discussed. Neither the author nor the publisher shall be liable or responsible for any loss or adverse effects allegedly arising from any information or suggestion in this book. While every effort has been made to ensure the accuracy of the information presented, neither the author nor the publisher assume any responsibility for errors.

This book is not intended to heal you. There is nothing medically proven or scientifically tested on these pages. This is merely my personal story with my autoimmune illness, Multiple Sclerosis, over the last 25 years and the various concepts, diets, routines, and exercises that I have followed. Not everything was easy; some of it was fun and creative, but in the end, it made me believe that I was doing something to take better care of myself while learning how to improve the health of my family at the same time.

My only hope for you, the reader, is to make you smile, pass a new idea onto you, or inspire you in some way. Personally I got tired of reading medical literature and wanted something that would uplift my spirits and yours. So keep an open mind, find some humour in my stories, and take the best care of yourself that you possibly can.

PERSONAL NOTE

Writing a book and sharing my story was harder than I thought it would be...I guess that's why it took me years to complete. It became a healing process that not only guided me, but gave me a personal goal and provided a creative daily routine. It started out as random pages for myself, to maybe pass onto my children, or a short story to reflect on. Then it became...this.

Dedication

To my remarkable children, Kean and Tatum,
who inspire me every day.

Table of Contents

Foreword

My first experience of Kelli was from a distance at our sons' basketball practices. I was seated in the gymnasium when I first saw Kelli enter with her cane in hand. With each step she took, she would swing her left leg forward as if it were a bag of rocks. Her gait appeared arduous and cumbersome.

In recognition of her physical impairment, my initial feelings were of compassion, but those feelings quickly changed to admiration as I observed her warm smile and optimistic nature as she greeted fellow parents.

Over the following months, I would continue to see Kelli at our sons' basketball games, and she always exuded such a positive demeanor. We eventually struck up a conversation and I discovered that she had a keen interest in natural healthcare. When Kelli and her family became patients at my chiropractic clinic, my admiration for them only grew. Caring for Kelli has afforded me the opportunity to experience her captivating spirit and witness her living life to the fullest, overcoming challenges like a champion. Her optimism, strength, and resolve are a joy to experience, and are key to the results she is able to achieve on a daily basis. To know Kelli is to know that she will not let her left leg hold her back; rather, she forces that leg to keep up with her.

Fabulous in Flats outlines Kelli's 25-year journey of discovery living with Multiple Sclerosis. It chronicles her ups and downs. It's a treasure trove of Kelli's experiences with her natural healthcare commitment and how it has optimized her health and happiness while minimizing the effects of Multiple Sclerosis on her lifestyle. Sprinkle in some of Kelli's lighthearted stories, and what you find in *Fabulous in Flats* is a great recipe to inspire, to enlighten, and to give hope to those who suffer physically or emotionally with chronic conditions of any nature.

Kelli may be *Fabulous in Flats*, but she lives her life as if she is in running shoes.

Rob Murray, DC
DOCTOR OF CHIROPRACTIC

Murray Family Chiropractic Clinic, Newmarket, Ontario
Founder of 360 Health — Lifestyle Management Workshops

Preface

Shoes, shoes, shoes. The choices are endless: pumps, kitten heels, sling backs, platforms, wedges, stilettos, t-straps, loafers, ballet flats.

I often get asked, "Where did you come up with the book title? Your book isn't about fashion or shoes..." Okay, I never get asked that question, but I wanted a reason to explain.

When does the love story between shoes and women really begin? As young girls the thought of playing dress up on a daily basis controls every waking thought. Probably around the age of three, girls begin to pretend to be a princess in a fancy gown, a ballet dancer in a tutu, or even a superhero with a cape. Acting out the characters while in costume creates joy for everyone in the house.

Shoes are usually the first object of desire for young girls. They watch Mom walk around, which shoes she puts on depending on the occasion, and imitate her expression and body language that changes with each step. Shoes offer kids the chance to feel grown up or like they're going to exciting places. They come in every color imaginable — some with peep toes, laces, buckles, bows, rhinestones, ankle straps, or beads.

This love affair never really ends. Shoes play an important role in life. As the years pass and every birthday comes along, a new series of rules is introduced. Age-appropriate styles, based on family beliefs, are introduced. The younger the girl, the flatter the shoe is. By grade 4 or 5, some height is introduced in sandals, boots, and dress shoes by either a wedge or traditional low heel. But as the years go by, the heels get taller and the projected image changes. It's both exciting and heartbreaking as a mother to watch the stages progress so quickly.

Shoes play an important role in women's psychology as well. The sensation of wearing high heels provides women with a desirable perception. High heels portray a status of power and beauty. They help women feel taller, create the illusion of longer legs, and provide a level of confidence, thus empowering women both professionally and socially. Self-image is very important and the perception of that image to the public is critical in a woman's mind.

Shoes participate in many of life's biggest events; the cute bow-tie pair for a grade school birthday party, the chunky heel for grade 8 graduation, the stiletto peep toe sandals to match your prom dress, the professional look for your first job, the romantic style to match your wedding gown, and the casual ones for your family life. Just as your life changes, so do your shoes and your love affair with them.

That brings me to the title of this book. As the progression of my illness has continued over the course of the last 25 years, my love affair has changed significantly with shoes. My desires and emotions around shoes had to evolve. No longer having the freedom to select high heels to match my pretty dress, I had to open my mind to view flat shoes as being sexy (still working on that). This was not easy. I missed the extra height, the length it added to my legs, the muscle definition, and the confidence (that I thought) they provided. Plus, I enjoy dressing fancy and high heels were a focal accessory in that process.

So my changes started out small. The heel height became lower over the years. Eventually the wide chunky heel was reintroduced (thank God I saved my Hushpuppies from the 90s). Then the wedge look was prominent for years, and now finally the flat shoe had to be the answer.

It was not easy, nor accepted by me in the beginning. I would continue to wear those damn heels, stumbling, hanging onto chairs, leaning against the walls, or anything I could grab — all while also clinging to my hope to continue to wear heels. I would even wear them to an event and at the first chance, remove them (Don't worry, I had a pedicure done!).

It is still not an easy option. Trust me, some (private) tears have been shed. I know, I know, they are only shoes. But they are so much more than that. It was the beginning of the end for many life choices that I would have to continue to adapt to. It was the knowledge that my illness was affecting me and everyone was going to notice.

It is 2023 now, and I am finally able to confidently say "I look *fabulous in flats.*" I shop for dressy flats, summer sandals, professional slip-ons, and comfortable boots. Nothing has really changed except for my comfort level.

So, go about your day feeling *fabulous*, with whatever fashion choices work for you.

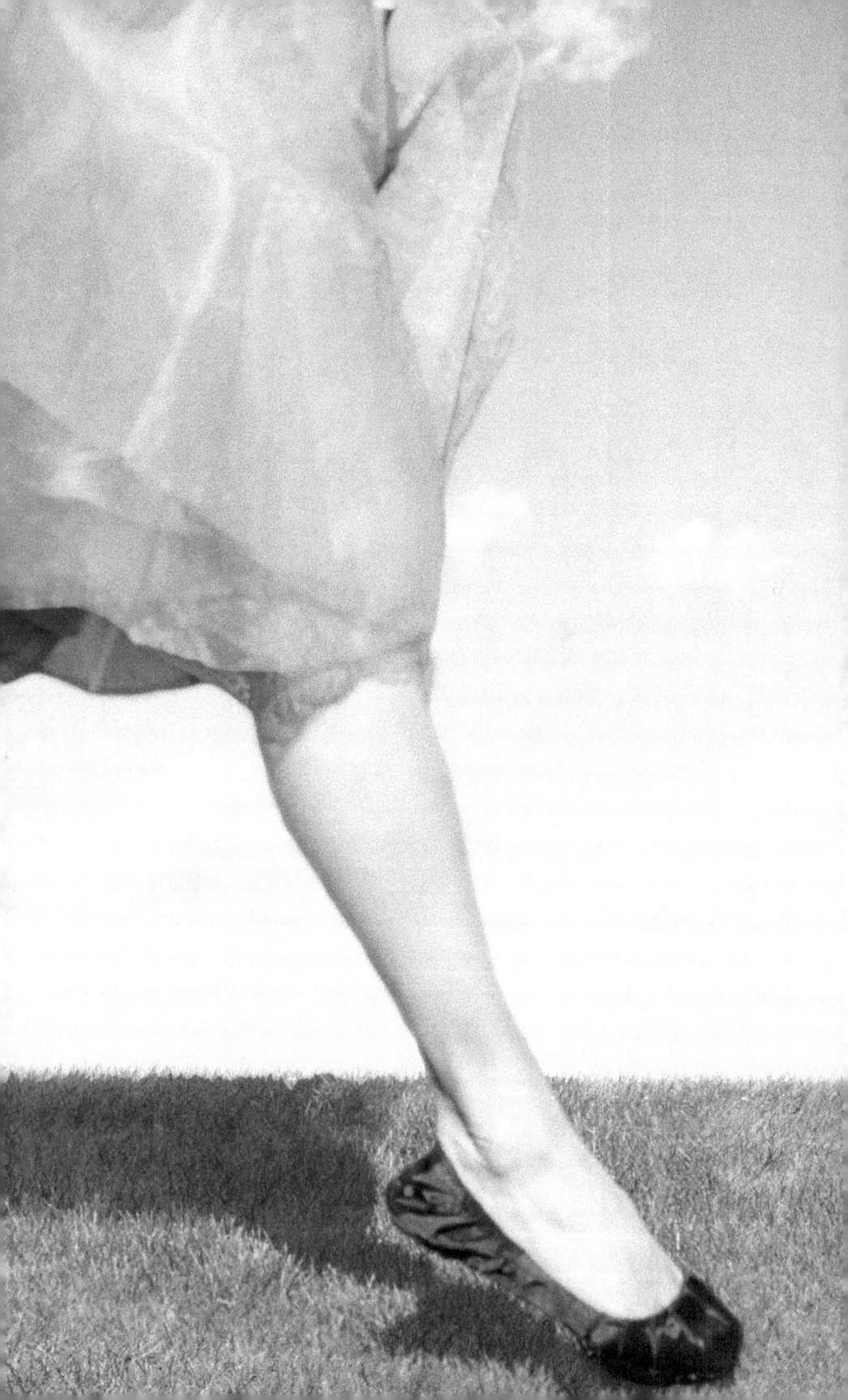

Part One

HERE WE ARE

Introduction

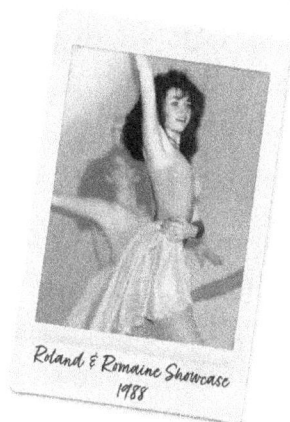

Roland & Romaine Showcase
1988

*M*y life has always revolved around dance. Ironically, my life journey was to involve an autoimmune illness that would limit the movement my body so craved.

I can remember going to dance lessons at a community centre when I was seven years old. I was good (or so my Brownie ribbon told me). After that, I attended a studio on Bloor Street in Toronto. I loved every minute of it, and even ended up being selected for the Kid Company (which, I have to say, you had to audition for, and in those days you had to patiently wait for an acceptance letter to come in the mail). Once accepted, it meant that I had to enroll in all of the dance categories offered: jazz, tap, ballet, ballroom, and musical theatre. This was long before competitive dance took over the world.

I spent most of my childhood at the studio. I performed in shows throughout the city, danced on the Sick Kids Telethon every year (look at me, I am on TV!) and even got some paying jobs. Then my true passion came; I became a teacher.

The studio became my life — and what a great life it was. I continued to teach for 20 years. I loved the studio, the owners, the teachers, the kids, the families, the deli upstairs, the pictures on the wall, the staff dressing room...basically everything. That studio and all of the people in it were my life. I should have taken more pictures. If only we had had cell phones back then to document memories like we do now.

Through dancing came fitness, and my interest in any kind of movement to strengthen, tone, or develop myself grew. I joined a gym, lifted weights, and flourished in aerobics classes. So, of course, I started teaching the super popular step classes of the '90s! Remember those? The music, the studio bursting with healthy bodies, the routines, the sweat...ahh, what great times.

Once college was completed, around age 21, I began working in the fashion industry for a Canadian designer. On top of working full time, teaching dance in the evenings and weekends for various dance studios and skating clubs, and leading aerobics classes at fitness centres, I also would exercise for myself as much as possible. It makes me tired just thinking about it. No wonder something had to give.

And it did!

MY LIFE AT AGE 24

Where to start? Where, oh where, to start? It feels like a lifetime ago, and it kind of is — twenty-five years ago, in a land far, far away...

The beginning is hard to remember, yet I have told my story over and over again throughout the years. Twenty-five years later (and learning to my surprise that I now have secondary progressive multiple sclerosis — WHAT?? — guess I didn't read that far into the medical books), I am sure I have forgotten half of the details. My memory is not that great anymore — which, by the way, has nothing to do with aging or wine consumption!

My life was really good in my 20s. I had a terrific group of friends, enjoyed going out dancing most weekends, and liked to host parties with my roommate. I found the man of my dreams, fell in love, we spent every waking moment together, and within a few months, he moved in. My family loved him, his family liked me (I think), and we were in heaven. The future was open. Anything we wanted to conquer was ours for the taking.

We had been dating for about a year when I began to notice interesting health issues popping up. It started slowly; it was hard to tell there was anything wrong with me. I just didn't feel right. I have always paid attention to my body and if something felt funny, I would research why.

It started with heart palpitations, so I was put on a device to monitor my heartbeat. Nothing came of that. Then one day, I noticed tingling down the back of my legs. My first thought was a pinched nerve, which happens all the time to physically active people. So I ignored it. After a while, I decided to visit the doctor, but she did not have any suggestions or answers.

The mystery would remain and my life would continue to move forward. No other symptoms ever came up, just the occasional tingling sensation. I did notice that it only happened upon standing up or the motion of looking down as you go to stand up. Weird. So I would sit and look down, tingling. Turn my head, no tingling. Look down, tingling. So yes, a pinched nerve for sure. This was before Google, so self-diagnosis was not as easy.

THE DIAGNOSIS

Off to the chiropractor I went, because of the supposed pinched nerve. He adjusted me, but that did not help. Then two phone calls took place later in the week. The chiropractor called and advised me to get a referral to see a neurologist. Then my GP doctor also called, and told me that she had referred me to see a neurologist. Okay, wait, what is a neurologist?

I was young, enjoying life, and did not have time to go to a hospital to talk to a new doctor. And at a hospital? No way. That is completely out of my comfort zone. I am a healthy 25-year-old woman.

WHAT IS GOING ON!?

I don't want to bore you with all of the details, so I am jumping ahead here. Of course the referral did not happen right away. I had to find a time to fit in the neurologist appointment around my numerous jobs. I was a very important person, and I didn't want to let any students down by missing a class (at least this is what I told myself).

On the day of my appointment, we traveled to the hospital (by we, I mean my handsome boyfriend and I). I had to complete routine laboratory tests and get an MRI (Magnetic Resonance Imaging) scan to confirm a medical diagnosis.

The MRI test (the first time) was fine. It is a large cylindrical-shaped tube surrounded by a circular magnetic machine.

As you lay on a moveable table that slides you into the centre of the tube, straps are placed around your wrists and across your forehead. There can be no movement for the duration of the test, which is usually 20–40 minutes. (I think. It has been a while and it seems I have blocked out those memories.) It is very loud, so you are given earplugs and/or headphones to communicate with the technician. I think that is supposed to calm and relax you. It doesn't.

Then the day finally came for me to return to my neurologist and receive the news. Actually, it might have all happened on the same day (again, blocked memories). I do remember sitting in her office and being told that the MRI scan confirmed that I had lesions on my brain, which meant that I have multiple sclerosis. I was diagnosed with relapsing-remitting MS (RRMS). Congratulations!

The nice (I did not like her right then) doctor handed me a pamphlet and explained that my version of MS would mean that I would have times when my symptoms would flare up, called relapses (so my tingling would get worse? Still not understanding), and then the attack or flare up would be followed by a time of recovery, where I would experience limited to no symptoms. (What are the symptoms? I really need to read the pamphlet.)

The name multiple sclerosis actually means multiple scars, and I had a few. Upon hearing this news, my life changed and a new journey began. Very, very rapidly.

Shock, confusion, numbness, fear, dread, loss, devastation, and questions...so many questions.

A NEW JOURNEY BEGINS

Apparently, my day was only beginning at the hospital. I was confused, upset, and felt like I was being directed around like a child. At this point, my mom joined us at the hospital to try to understand what was happening.

I was advised to join a research program for a new drug that was being tested. I agreed to learn more — (did I have a choice? I still hadn't read the pamphlet) — and had to travel to meet with a different doctor at another hospital in the city. So basically, pay for parking again!

I still had no idea at this point what MS really was or how it was going to affect my life. Every emotion was running through me and I had a dance class to teach at 4:30 p.m., so I had to get to work. How long would this take?

A family decision was made after meeting with a new neurologist (with terrible bedside manner, to say the least) and I joined a research program. This then started my new lifelong fear of needles! Can't get them, can't watch anyone else getting them, and don't even like to talk about them. But I will try to recreate the humor that was involved on a weekly basis surrounding them.

Medicine is a strange principle to me. Doctors and nurses study for numerous years to perfect their craft, and yet my boyfriend was trained, with the use of an orange, how to insert an intramuscular (code word for painful) needle into various locations on my body. Not only that, but we had to learn how to mix the drug and put the correct amount in the syringe. We were trained so that we could do everything ourselves at home — wasn't that nice of them?

The drug I was placed on was either the real deal or a placebo. I had no idea. All I knew was that three times a week, in different locations, my boyfriend was going to insert a very long, sharp needle into one of my muscles. He had to use the correct amount of force to get through the muscle (gross thought) and gently release the liquid from the syringe. This created a lot of tension for both of us. I hated getting them and he hated giving them. But I was lucky; the drug (or placebo) was free. Did you read that right? I was being put through this torture with the possibility of receiving a liquid that has no curative effect. Nothing, zero, zilch. And the only good news was that it was free.

So I participated in the research program, received the needle three times a week, continued to work full-time, taught dance in the evenings, and enjoyed life.

Then the various symptoms started to arrive, just like the pamphlet said. (I did get around to reading it.) I think I experienced most of them: vision problems, numbness in hands, tightness of ribs, leg numbness, foot dragging, dizziness, bladder problems (don't get me started on that one), stiff muscles, feeling weak/tired, balance problems, and various emotional symptoms.

They were confusing, annoying, and all I wanted was something to make them go away. I enjoyed keeping busy. In the beginning it did not stop me unless it was a bad flare up. And even then, I would push through it. I remember numerous times teaching my dance class while sitting. I participated in the local MS walks and raised money for research. I read every book I could get my hands on and tried to stay positive.

I am not sure when the research program stopped, or if my doctor took me off of it in order to now prescribe a real MS drug for me to take. Thankfully, I had health insurance so a portion of the cost was covered. We still had a good chunk to pay, though, because those drugs are not cheap.

The drug was really no better. Still a stupid needle, folks. The (false) hope that it would make everything go away, and then months later I would have a flare-up again, was defeating. It was exhausting.

Over the years, many funny stories (only funny now, 25 years later) took place. The drugs (steroids) to deal with symptoms were always entertaining as I would have the energy of a hummingbird beating its wings non-stop. I could not sleep, would move from bed to couch, back to the bed and kick my boyfriend out again, only to return back to the couch. This lasted for hours during the night.

The lack of sleep was not helping my body heal or my mind to remain focused on daily activities. This would go on for days until the steroids would start to take effect. Then the withdrawal symptoms would start. It was an endless time of torture, only to be followed by months (hopefully) of recovery.

Honestly, we laugh at these stories remembering what we went through. The drugs came to an end for me — no more needles or steroids about three years from that fateful day in the neurologist's office. I decided to go off the drug and explore a different approach. I was able to surround myself with holistic doctors, therapists, and wonderful natural health providers who guided me to research, educate, and change my life in ways that I never could have imagined.

The inspiring message about my story is that I am healthy, living a full life, and have found strategies to deal with my illness. I am grateful every day for what I have in my life, all of the activities I can still participate in, and everyone who encourages me to never give up.

Whether you are also battling MS, have an autoimmune illness, or are just looking to learn, I hope that something I share catches your eye or makes you think about a new concept to add to your health regimen. Stay strong and be... *fabulous*.

1

Having an Illness SUCKS!

*Y*es, you heard that right. I am not going to sugar coat it or try to inspire you in this section (well, maybe). Having a chronic illness that you can never heal SUCKS! Your life will never be the same. Your future will be unknown. Blah, blah, blah.

Life sometimes sucks, period. Your issues might be health, wealth, love, illness, or family members. But the end result is all about how you deal with it, control it, or give in to it. Not giving in is very hard and takes time.

FIVE REASONS WHY BEING SICK SUCKS

The Unknown

I have WHAT? Pardon me? What's that? Huh?

Being diagnosed is both the relieving aspect and hardest part. Do I really want to know what is wrong? Will I feel relief or anger, judgment, or disbelief from the actual knowledge of my health?

I lived with symptoms, never understanding what was making me feel the way I did, and experienced relief when I was told that I could have some testing done. Phew! Now I can get the answers and everything will be fine! For me, everything happened so fast — the hospital, the MRI scan, and the diagnosis. Way too much for a 25-year-old to handle or even comprehend. Everything was not FINE.

Now the guessing game began. I had no idea when my symptoms would change, go away, or resurface. Will a drug help me? Will it make me feel worse? How much does it cost? The funny thing about being young, though, is that it never fully registered with me. (I thought I was invincible.) I figured the medical world would help me every step of the way. This illness would not really affect me. *How could it?* If I have a flare up, I'll take steroids and feel better. Nothing a pill can't cure. Living with the unknown is an emotional roller coaster.

The Invisible Side

Everyone walks around with a mask on. We never truly understand what is happening within other people's lives. God forbid you find out and learn that they are human. We are so good at hiding how we are feeling, it almost seems normal.

It took me years to be able to feel comfortable communicating to people about my illness simply because I don't *look* sick. (Well, that's a lie; I still get emotional telling people, as my voice cracks or I look away.) In the beginning you could tell that there was something wrong as my flare ups affected my hands so my writing was messy, or I sat in a chair to teach dance because my legs were weak, or I was just crying at my desk wondering when this would end.

As a result, I didn't want to go out. I chose not to socialize during a flare-up because I was worried about what other people would think of me — or even how they would look at me. On the outside, I looked healthy. You could not tell that I was having any symptoms unless you were a close friend, family member, or I told you. I never faked being sick; I faked being well.

The capacity to hide has become so easy. As long as I'm sitting, my makeup is on, my hair is styled, my clothes are fashionable (no yoga pants), and I am smiling...I must be having a good day. People have no idea that I am stressed out, my left hand is numb, walking is an extreme chore, and I need to use the bathroom right now!

The Unpredictability of Every Day

I am a planner. I always have been and always will be. Living with an illness has only magnified this special skill. The unpredictability of everyday life is a well thought out, researched, planned, and emotional existence that I have to try to manipulate so I have everything under control.

Personally, I have to plan every movement of every day so that I don't get stressed (wait, isn't all that planning stressful, too?). No surprises or last minute changes can be added to my calendar. Never knowing how I am going to feel upon waking, after eating, finishing my shower, the weather forecast, how tired an activity will make me, and remembering to rest are all taken into account.

If I plan to attend a sporting/dance event, I have to figure out and/or allow time to: walk to the car (both at home and at the venue), map out the driving route with bathroom stops (again, taking into account the time this takes up), what the temperature is both inside and outside the venue (too hot and I melt, too cold and I freeze), what the entrance is like (stairs, ramps, elevators), what the distance is from the main door to the final destination, where the bathroom is inside the venue (again with the bathrooms), the seating availability, the event duration, where and when food will be available, and how long it will take to get home.

Some events I just can't attend; it is too difficult and I end up exhausting myself for the next two days to recuperate. Those are the hardest to deal with because I don't want to miss out on participating in these life experiences. Accepting this takes years and I still work on it daily. I hate the thought of letting anyone down or looking weak, but then I remember that I have an autoimmune illness and anything that I can still do is to be acknowledged (even if just by myself). I am grateful each day for what I can participate in. It helps to try not to focus on what I have missed.

The Things You Give Up

Living with any autoimmune illness is an emotional rollercoaster. One day you have the energy of a racehorse and want to get out into the world. Other days you can barely get out of bed or off of the couch. Then there are so many days where you watch your family participate in activities that you no longer can and smile (Oscar-winning performance) and encourage them not to miss out on anything due to you.

The loss of engaging in life events can be all-consuming. I want to run, dance, take my kids out, participate in adventures, ride a bike, socialize, and go for long walks with my family. I enjoy being busy; I don't like sitting around wasting time. That just creates more stress. So I jump up (well, slowly move to the edge of the couch, rise up, stand still to allow my muscles to prepare to move, maybe reach for the wall) and take a step forward. I have to stay focused on the task and work diligently so I am optimizing my energy.

I remind myself every day that I have not given anything up. I have had to learn to recognize what I can't do, accept it, and then do what I can — just differently. The days take more planning, more discipline, and more patience, but they are still filled with love and life.

The Future

The future is unknown for everybody, illness or not. I just have to think about where my illness "might" be in my future. I try to stay positive and work towards it remaining relatively the same. One thing that has helped has been to arrange my surroundings to better suit my needs. I have updated my shower so that it is a walk-in style, our patio chairs all have arm rests so that I can use them to push up from, furniture has been moved to create a more open space for my movement, and storage has been added on the main level instead of keeping supplies in the basement.

Having a chronic illness really does suck, but I work to deal with it the best way I can. I try to live in the present moment and enjoy everything in my life. The fridge calendar is essential, not only for my memory but for planning what is coming up. I have two energetic teenagers who keep me busy and I love every minute of it. My participation looks different, but I make sure that I am attending every event I can.

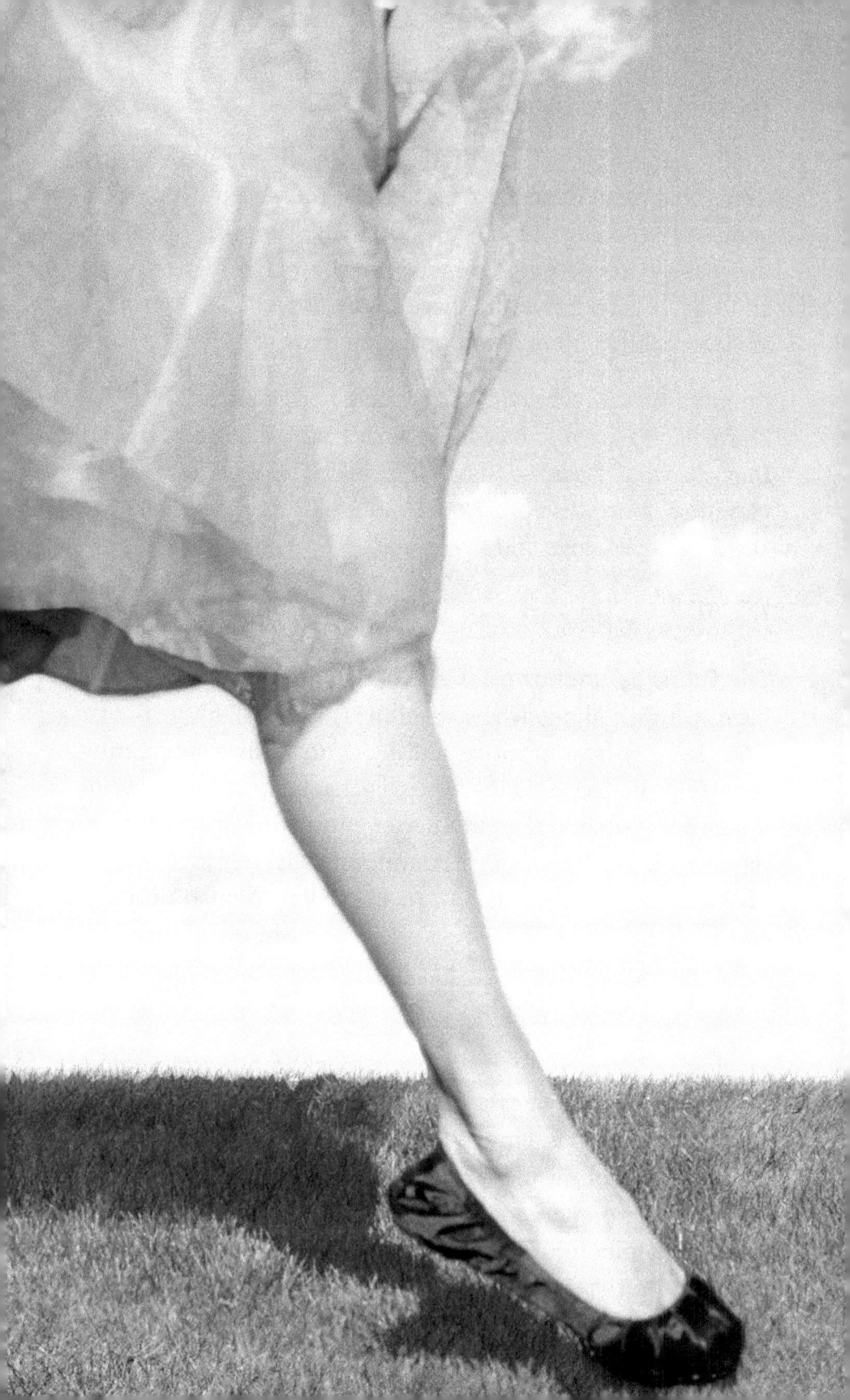

Part Two

HEALTH

2

Holistic Medicine: My Journey Into the Unknown

Having an autoimmune illness has brought about so many learning curves, experiences, expectations, and confusion for me over the years. Along the way I have had the privilege to meet incredible people who have truly changed my life and opened up my mind. Holistic Medicine includes treatments that can benefit, and even complement, traditional therapies.

My plan is to have a toolkit of practitioners to help create the best future I can. The list of options are endless but I am just going to concentrate on the natural practitioners that I have tried, learned from, and continue to follow on a regular basis.

MASSAGE THERAPY

Who doesn't love to get a massage? The impact alone of physical touch on our brain is profound. Massage used to be considered a luxury and indulgence for some; spending the afternoon at an expensive spa, sipping on a fruit-filled beverage, and relaxing in a cozy robe. Okay, maybe I watch too many movies.

I was very lucky in my early diagnosis as I was referred to the most loving, spiritual, healing, and incredible massage therapist I have ever met. But it wasn't just the actual massage that was fantastic, it was the entire experience she provided.

She practiced out of her 2-bedroom apartment in Toronto. The decor was tranquil, essential oils filled the air, and the cat that always came over to greet you along with the open door and gracious welcome made it feel like home. She would spend time with you before and after, just talking, telling you all about her life and wanting to learn everything about yours.

She became a true friend. She would offer guidance, helpful advice, and any suggestions to help me in my healing. She was even a guest at my wedding, and we still smile every year when we watch the video. She loved to dance and was on the dance floor the whole time.

Now in 2023, massage therapy is a lucrative business. It is offered in spas, health clubs, nail salons, hair salons, wellness clinics, and in private home businesses. There is a good reason for this: everyone is stressed out. You see it everywhere you look: in the faces of co-workers, in the grocery store clerks, on the bus, and at your dinner table.

The benefits of massage are too extensive to list in full. I will highlight the basics, and the areas that really resonate with me.

1) Relieves stress
2) Reduces anxiety
3) Reduces muscle tension
4) Improves sleep
5) Improves joint stiffness

The list goes on and on regarding the benefits. It is worth looking into. Find someone you trust and spoil yourself!

HOMEOPATHY

Ahh, just the word brings a sense of calm for me. The history of homeopathy begins with discoveries that were made over 200 years ago. It is based on the principle of the law of similars, essentially treating "like with like" — meaning that a substance that causes a reaction when taken in large doses can be used in smaller doses to treat those exact symptoms.

Again, this can be a confusing topic and one met with resistance. It has really grown in popularity since I was introduced to it. And back then, it took a while for me to even consider it! I had no prior introduction to it.

Back to that fantastic massage therapist I just told you about. She had started talking to me about a homeopathic doctor that she knew and felt he could really help with my MS symptoms. For months I let her talk, agreeing or nodding my head, while not really listening or considering finding out more. Finally it must have started to make sense (or I just really wanted to get her to stop mentioning him) so I booked an appointment to meet this doctor. I didn't know at the time that it would change my life.

So off I went. My boyfriend even came with me because I was too nervous to go alone. The office was quiet, the receptionist was his wife, and he had red hair! I knew I would like him for that fact alone, being a redhead myself. It was an easy conversation. He made me feel very comfortable, put my fears at ease, and told me he could help me with my symptoms. WHAT? Just that positive statement alone felt wonderful.

So I put my trust in him and have never looked back.

In the early days, when I would have a flare up (numbness), the doctor would prescribe steroids for me to take. They always affected me for days, and I never truly felt like myself. Eventually they would wear off and my symptoms would be gone. I hated taking them but felt that there were no other options.

Now, I had homeopathy on my side and I started this journey by taking a remedy to help with the numbness. Guess what? It worked! And with no side effects or sleepless nights.

Twenty-five years later, this doctor is still my savior in my MS journey. I have appointments every month to stay on a schedule and keep my body healthy. He has been with me every step of the way. He witnessed me getting married, having children, changing jobs, moving, treating my kids as they have grown up, and has watched me become an advocate for homeopathy.

Having worked with a doctor for twenty-five years is a blessing that I can't even explain. Hell, I've known him, or should I say, he has known me, for as long as my husband has. I can't hide anything from him. He just refers back to my files (paper files) to confirm or compare symptoms.

In our house we use homeopathy for everything and everyone, even the dog. Remedies are inexpensive and can be found at most natural stores.

CHIROPRACTIC MEDICINE

This complementary medical practice has a long history: over 100 years, in fact. The basic chiropractic principle is to apply techniques or adjustments that align your spine and body structure to improve overall function, ease pain, and allow your body to heal itself naturally.

Basically, the spine is our nervous system which affects every part of the body. It is responsible for all movement, organ functions, and even our five senses (sight, sound, touch, taste, and smell). This system carries all information to the brain so that it can process and help the body react appropriately. If the spine is not aligned or is out of balance, it can impact the function of the nervous system, creating pain, decreasing mobility, and compromising our immune system. Not only the spine can be adjusted; the legs, hips, or arms might need to be aligned as well.

What I like about chiropractors is the personal touch and the authentic interest in your overall health. They treat you and your unique personal symptoms, they get to know you, they ask questions, and they offer additional health advice.

Fast-forward to my life now. The first doctor my family visits when any health symptoms appear is our chiropractor. My kids go and have been going ever since they were a few days old. Whether it is a runny nose, stuffed up nose, growing pains, sports injury, ankle issues from dance, headache, stomach ache, cough, congestion, sore throat, or neck pain, we all get adjusted. Our immune system has been compromised and needs to get back into balance.

Within a day or two, the symptoms have improved, if not completely disappeared. And I didn't need to wait in a crowded, germ-infested waiting room to be given a prescription for a pill. We are not rushed through our appointment. We talk about our weekend. We share family stories and have a laugh with the receptionist as we leave.

REFLEXOLOGY

Are you ticklish? Do you have sensitive feet? Well, I do, too. Reflexology involves applying pressure to specific areas on the feet, hands, or ears. It's kind of like a massage for the extremities. I have only ever had it performed on my feet. Trust me, "dancer's feet" are ugly, so I was embarrassed at first.

The idea is that areas of the foot correspond to different body organs and systems. It has the ability to positively affect a person's overall health. Applying pressure to a specific location on the arch of the foot could benefit bladder function (I even apply essential oils to the pressure points).

I lucked out again! I was referred to an extraordinary reflexologist who played a key role in my healing in the early stages. She worked out of her beautiful home and created the caring environment that I needed. Needless to say, she also came to my wedding.

TRADITIONAL CHINESE MEDICINE (TCM)

I began to incorporate acupuncture into my health regimen in 2019. Honestly, I was nervous about the needles — tiny, sterile needles that are inserted about half an inch or even less into specific points on the body. Seriously, that is what I was anxious about.

Acupuncture is virtually painless and can be extremely relaxing. Traditional Chinese Medicine has been used in China for thousands of years to not only fight disease but prevent it. It is believed that vital energy, "Qi," flows through the body and if there is a blockage or imbalance of Qi, then pain and illness is created. Acupuncture needles gently encourage the body to restore the balance and the flow of energy.

I did my research and found a wonderful TCM Practitioner. With his family history of the practice and having studied in China, I was confident for my first appointment. This was important to me. I wanted to know that I had the best before I let anyone put needles (again, they are tiny) into my skin.

My appointments help with all my symptoms: anxiety, bladder function, balance, dizziness, and pain. We spend time discussing my symptoms, looking at my tongue, applying pressure to my muscles, feeling for any heat in my hands or feet, and assessing where my mental state is — usually anxious — before I lay down.

Once the needles are inserted, he lowers the lights and leaves the room. This allows me to relax (as best I can). The time goes by quickly before he returns and removes the needles. We chat, and he advises me on what improvements to watch for and what exercises I can perform at home.

OSTEOPATHY

Manual Osteopathy is another holistic form of hands-on therapy that I enjoy. It is different from chiropractic as it focuses on joint movements, stretching the muscles, soft tissue massage, muscle resistance techniques, and the body's nervous system. The treatments are mostly manipulation of the body to bring it back to a healthy state.

I try to attend monthly sessions where we work on relieving any pain that I might have, reducing joint stiffness in my hips, increasing circulation, decreasing inflammation, increasing my range of motion, strengthening my ankles, and encouraging my body to heal itself. The specific stretches work perfectly, as they are hard to complete on your own (especially when you have trouble getting up from the floor).

The initial benefits can be hard to measure. It is normal to experience some mild soreness in the treatment area. Even though it is a gentle technique, it is still a workout for me. My body doesn't usually do that much movement for a solid hour on a regular day.

I enjoy osteopathy, as I feel that it helps me to develop a healthier lifestyle. It's another tool that I use to restore my body, increase healing, and get me out of the house.

PHYSIOTHERAPY

It took me a long time to incorporate a physical therapist into my healing program. I assumed that they were only necessary for injuries, accidents, or surgery recovery. Never understanding — or rather, misunderstanding — how a PT could help me, I am new to this approach. Having had my fitness background, this treatment feels like having my own personal fitness trainer.

Working with a physical therapist involves learning functional exercises to help strengthen muscles, strategies to improve energy, and techniques to deal with various mobility issues. The treatments or sessions help to restore, maintain, and guide you on how to function with your illness. Exercise is so important for reducing inflammation, improving immune function, enhancing brain structure, reducing fatigue, and increasing oxygen supply to your brain.

My appointments are actually fun and social. We work on my current level of mobility, identify issues, and develop a plan to improve any weaknesses. Exercises are repeated, weights are lifted, and my confidence in my abilities is restored. I am encouraged to practice at home and continue to strengthen my body until next time.

I am always researching any form of natural healing that might help me with my symptoms. It sounds like I do a lot, all the time. I don't! Having a schedule that I can change, alter, add, or reduce when needed is what works for me. Life with a family and work takes over and appointments get missed. But that's okay. That is a part of my care; some days run smoothly, some don't.

25 OF THE BEST THINGS THAT I DID FOR MYSELF

1) I created an office space and not a spare room that junk gathers in.

2) I consume a glass of warm lemon water each morning. It aids in digestion, rehydration, and reduces inflammation.

3) We invested in a gas fireplace for the basement. Not only does it produce heat, but it creates a cozy atmosphere for relaxation and tranquility while I do yoga.

4) We renovated the main bathroom to make it a walk-in shower.

5) I purchased a carpet to go under the bed, over the beautiful hardwood floor. Now my feet stay warm as they touch down from the cozy blanket in the morning.

6) I journal gratitude each morning and practice meditation.

7) I schedule time each day for exercise — no excuses. 30 minutes is all I need.

8) I began to study essential oils and learn the healing benefits they provide.

9) I limited the processed baked goods and began to bake (no gluten, no dairy) treats instead.

10) I aligned myself with some wonderful and inspiring social media leaders. I kicked the Facebook friend following habit (nothing personal) and added health leaders to follow instead.

11) I began to grocery shop online and pick-up, all while staying in the car.

12) I kicked the habit of stressing over cooking and went back to the basics of nutrition at every meal: a protein portion, colorful vegetables, a salad, some fruit, and water.

13) I set up a weekly delivery from a local farmer. Veggies never tasted so good!

14) I purchased a Red Light Therapy device to use every morning.

15) I made the decision to get adult braces. Finally straightening my teeth feels fantastic.

16) I continue to book my treatments regularly. I set up a care plan, commit to appointments, and show up.

17) I ended the cycle of matching my eating pattern to whomever I am with. Instead, I choose the food that reflects my health beliefs: no gluten, no dairy, more greens.

18) I celebrate my daily successes.

19) I no longer answer my phone/text every time it chirps. When I am prepared and focused, I will respond.

20) I set a reading goal for the year of 16 books. Some years it's more, some years it's less.

21) I made a conscious decision to let my kids be bored! No, I will not entertain you. Go outside or create something for yourself to do (and I will not feel guilty).

22) I encouraged the children's social time with friends. They can hang out, play video games, and spend time TOGETHER!

23) I took my dog to daycare. The pure joy and excitement he demonstrates from the suggestion of this weekly event brings laughter into the house.

24) I witnessed the effects of paying it forward on a regular basis. I truly believe that what you put into the universe will come back to you.

25) I wrote this list! It reminds me of how amazing life is.

Now go write your own list of the best 25 things you have done for yourself!

3

Homeopathy

*Y*ou have probably heard of homeopathy, tried out a remedy such as arnica, or know someone who can't shut up about the healing benefits it provides. I am one of those annoying homeopathy promoters!

You've read a bit about my story and my introduction to homeopathy in previous sections of the book, but do you honestly know what the heck homeopathy is? It has taken me years to fully understand, incorporate, and be able to explain the holistic benefits it provides. It has really grown in popularity over the last twenty-five years since I was first introduced to it. And back then, it took a while for me to even consider it. I had no experience with homeopathy.

Essentially, it is a medical practice that uses tiny amounts of natural substances, like plants, food, and minerals, to stimulate the healing process in the body. Yes, stimulate, not suppress. That is a different approach than conventional medicine and opposite to what people think of when they are sick. Stimulating my cold?

Homeopaths depend on the remedies evoking a reaction from our immune system. The belief behind homeopathy is that "like cures like." What this means is that something that brings on symptoms in a healthy person can — in a very small dose — treat an illness in someone with similar symptoms. This will trigger the body's natural defense system. Homeopathy is the belief that the body has the ability to heal itself.

Confused yet? Imagine cutting an onion and your eyes start to water. A homeopathic remedy for allergies will contain onions as a treatment for the symptom of watery eyes.

Homeopathy is a system that follows three basic principles: the law of similars (like cures like), minimum dose, and a single remedy. Depending on what dosage and which remedy the doctor gives you, you only need one. You might just take two pellets and book a follow-up appointment in a month, or take pellets at a four-hour interval, or even take a remedy three times a day for a month. It all depends on the potency and your symptoms.

The other interesting aspect of homeopathy is that it not only deals with symptoms that you might be experiencing at a specific time, but also your mental, emotional, and physical health in total. It looks at the big picture of your health, from head to toe and from start to finish. Just think about the last time you had a head cold. Were you angry, exhausted, and emotional? Did you have body aches, chills, mucus, worsening symptoms at night, dry cough, loose cough...or did it have hardly any affect on you at all, other than a headache? How symptoms show up determines the best remedy for you. Your treatment is tailored to *you*. It's common for two patients with the same condition to receive different treatments.

The initial appointment can be a surprising experience. It is about two hours long, and you have to fill out pages and pages of questions about yourself and your family's health history, going back as far as you can remember, long before any of the recent symptoms you are experiencing began. The doctor needs to learn your whole story and why your health has undergone the changes to reflect your current state of well-being (or lack thereof). It can be daunting, overwhelming, and emotional. You really reflect on yourself. When was the last time that you thought or talked only about yourself for two hours?

Homeopathy was introduced to me at the right time in my life. I was open to learning (well, kind of), working with a new doctor, and stopping the treacherous cycle of painful needles with a drug that I was, personally, not seeing results from. I am so thankful to have found this holistic health approach for both myself and eventually for my family.

Living in our world today, choosing any holistic health practice is easy for me. Homeopathy allowed me to learn, feel like I have some control, build an inventory of remedies in my house, and take care of my family's health with knowledge and confidence.

Over the years, I have acquired basic remedies that work for common illnesses that pop up. While our first instinct (especially as parents) may be to purchase over-the-counter medications to resolve complaints, there are often natural remedies that don't interfere with the body's own immune system and can help ease uncomfortable symptoms.

Please note that I am not a doctor, so this section is for informational purposes only and is not intended to be used as a replacement when medical attention is needed! If you are new to homeopathy, it would be wise to seek out a homeopathic professional for any serious or chronic illnesses.

For acute situations, the following list of my basic remedies offers some simple and effective remedy suggestions to help you initially.

Calendula Cream

This is a fantastic remedy that incorporates antiseptic and antimicrobial actions that speed up the healing of wounds, minor cuts, relieves insect bites, acne, and is great on diaper rash. If you are allergic to plants, though, you will want to test the cream prior to layering it on your skin.

Arnica (30C)

I carry this remedy in my purse at all times! It can be used for any kind of trauma to the body (sports/dance for my kids), as well as muscle pain, head injuries, growing pains, or bruises. It is great for any pain after dental procedures, too.

Chamomilla (30C)

You've probably heard of the calming effects of chamomile tea. This remedy works wonders for teething babies and sleepless moms.

Pulsatilla (30C)

Think ear infections and thick green discharge. Key symptoms are emotional and tearful. I use this when there is goop in the eyes, coming out of the nose, or tears flowing!

Sulphur (30C)

Saturday night FEVER! Sweaty, hot, and red. Check that the hands, feet, and core body are all hot for the selection of this remedy.

Belladonna (30C)

High fever remedy. This is a dry, radiating temperature that comes on suddenly with intense heat. You will notice that the face is flushed with glazed eyes while the hands and feet remain cool. Belladonna also works for sunstroke with the same symptoms. It is a summer remedy in this house for all the redheads.

Spongia (30C)

Who let the dogs in? When the cough is loud, dry, and hoarse and sounds like a dog barking, spongia might help (think croup). Often there is a rasping respiration quality that creates difficulty for breathing. And of course this often happens during the night when you are all sleeping. An added note for this frantic situation: fresh, cold air helps to open the airways. In the winter, stand outside for ten minutes, taking deep breaths. You can even open the freezer and breathe in the cold air. You will notice that the breathing becomes normal and the coughing might even stop. This gives you time to prepare for any next steps to consider if needed.

Note: The remedies suggested will include a "30C" recommendation, which is the potency of the remedy.

Learning a little homeopathy can go a long way in easing your mind and nervous system when dealing with a virus. These are just a selection of my favorite remedies that have been valuable to have on hand for any situation that unexpectedly pops up. I provided basic symptoms but they offer support for so much more. It will give you time to consider all the options and what medical moves to make next.

FINDING HUMOUR IN LIFE

*L*ife is hard, folks. Everywhere, people are overstressed, overworked, underpaid, and overtired. It can be really hard to find anything funny about day-to-day life, whether you have an illness or are completely healthy. In today's world, people don't even notice those around them, let alone share a smile with a stranger. Most of the time, I don't want to be noticed or stand out in any way.

But I like to talk to people when I go out. It can be surprising to some, a waste of time to others, and embarrassing for my kids. I usually start a conversation in the grocery line with the mom and baby behind me, compliment another on her outfit, or say thank you to the building cleaner at the dance studio who does a great job keeping the stairs slip-free (a fact that is very important to me).

I have to share some recent interactions with you. They could have annoyed me, but I looked at them knowing that people are dealing with their own personal issues and doing their best to survive.

While walking in the grocery store, a fellow female shopper noticed that I was limping, so she asked:

Her: *"What happened? Did you hurt yourself?"*
Me: *"No, I didn't fall or anything, but thanks for asking. I have MS, so I tend to limp."*
Her: *"OMG, so do I. How long have you been a migraine sufferer? What do you take?"*

Okay, stop laughing! This was funny to me. I do get migraine headaches, so I just said Tylenol. No need to correct her or point out that was not what I meant. She was reaching out and sharing a part of herself, even if it had nothing to do with my situation. There was no harm done. It just reminded me that people are kind and she wanted to chat.

Exiting the bathroom at my son's basketball game, a gracious mom held the door open for me and asked:

Her: *"You are walking with a limp?"*
Me: *"Yes, I have MS and it affects my left leg."*
Her: *"I know the feeling. What other menopause symptoms do you have?"*

Again, stop shaking your head! I did not realize that limping was a side effect of menopause. This made me smile.

A delivery man arrived at my house, and while opening the door, I lost my balance (trying to open the door, hold the door, my cane, and remain standing at the same time). I fell right into the UPS driver's arms. He was mortified, scared, and did not find it amusing. He dropped the box, needless to say, and took off as soon as he could. Now deliveries just get left at my door.

Life is about laughing and living. Everyone means well and is at least starting a conversation — especially now with all of the technology keeping everyone so plugged in. It is rare to find someone not holding a cell phone, texting at rapid speeds, or with ear buds playing their favourite song. You think people are looking at you when you get off balance and stumble or drop your keys, but they don't see you. So don't worry about it!

4

Essential Oils

*B*y now, you know that I am very holistic-minded, and natural solutions are what I gravitate towards for myself and my family's health. So essential oils make sense, but initially they were comparable to potpourri for me — something my Grandmother put out to fragrance her house.

Then I attended a health training event where the presenter was using an essential oil diffuser in the room and it made me curious! Okay, let me backtrack a bit. Yes, I have experienced essential oils in yoga classes (loved it), at massages, in various stores, and at friends' homes, but it never really interested me or caught my attention from a health perspective before. What changed was the fact that it could be used for so much more than just in a diffuser.

Why it took me so long to figure out that I could include oils in my daily life to help with autoimmune symptoms, the yearly cold, inflammation, my mental well-being, and to consume internally, I will never know. I use essential oils every day now, in every room in the house, and on everyone. Honestly, I can't live without them.

In the beginning, I was completely unaware of any health benefits the oils are able to provide. I assumed you purchased fun scented blends, added drops to the diffuser, and walked away. Being a cheap, thrifty, economical (whatever descriptive word fits) shopper, I believed it wasn't worth spending $35+ on a 15ml bottle of a fragrance to be misted into the air. I would only purchase oils if they were on sale, in large bottles, or from Amazon. Honestly, I wasted a lot of time and money. I needed something different — something that empowered me.

It's been a few years of research on actual health benefits, watching YouTube videos, experimenting with oils, and I have fallen in love (read: *obsessed*) with oils. (Great! Another thing for me to spend money on!) I prefer doTERRA oils due to the quality, the discount, and the detailed education the company provides. Once I compared the results — and I witnessed them quickly — there was no turning back. The amount of websites on Google can be overwhelming, so deciding on a specific brand helped me keep it simple.

ESSENTIAL OILS 101

Essential oils are natural compounds found in the roots, stems, leaves, seeds, bark, flowers, and other parts of plants. They have been used throughout history and in many different cultures for their incredible healing properties, benefits, and therapeutic effects.

Therapeutic grade oils are most commonly created using low-heat steam distillation that captures their essence and oils. Once the product cools and separates, the oils are collected. One of the most important points to look for in your oils is that they are Certified Pure Therapeutic Grade (CPTG). This means they are 100 percent pure and contain no artificial fillers, aromas, chemicals, pesticide residues, or other harmful ingredients that would dilute their active healing properties. The quality of the oil definitely matters.

HAVE FUN WITH OILS

I have become addicted to essential oils and the unlimited benefits they provide. Not only do they help support and protect the body, they also ease common ailments such as headaches, muscle pain, anxiety, depression, digestion, concentration, incontinence, and so much more.

Now the fun and your creativity starts. Find the best way for you to experience all of the different uses that essential oils offer. Topically (on your body) is the quickest route for stimulating the health boosting benefits of the oils. Or, using a diffuser, you can mix oils with water and fill your entire living space with the scent. Even consuming specific oils internally by adding a few drops to a beverage or meals is a wonderful way to incorporate oils into your life.

HERE ARE DIFFERENT APPROACHES TO ENJOYING YOUR OILS:

Roller Bottles

Roller bottles or droppers are the perfect way to mix up your own essential oil blends. They make topical application of oils super simple, plus they can save you time and money. The roller ball on top will distribute the mixture onto whatever it touches, making it easy to apply just the right amount to the location of your choice. They're small enough that they won't take up much space in your purse, your car, or bedside table.

I prefer to use amber bottles with stainless steel metal roller balls when making my own. They roll much smoother than plastic rollerballs. To make your own, fill the bottle ¾ of the way up with carrier oil (e.g. fractionated coconut oil, jojoba oil, or almond oil), then add 10-15 drops of essential oil(s) to the roller bottle. Put the cap back on, roll the bottle between your palms to mix, and voila! Keep it simple. Use more or less essential oils depending on your preference.

Spray (Mist) Bottles

Misting the space surrounding you is another great way to enjoy essential oils. Think of it as your own personal air freshener. Keep a bottle at your desk, in your car, and in every room of the house. They can be used to freshen the air, disinfect a surface, improve your mood, enhance relaxation, increase concentration, and heighten feelings of joy and peace. The uses are endless.

I choose to use 4 oz. amber mist bottles for daily needs, and 16 oz. large spray bottles for my cleaning spray, bug spray, or disinfectant.

When creating my 4 oz. bottle, I start by adding 2 tablespoons of witch hazel (for preservation), 20-30 drops of your preferred oil(s), and fill the rest with distilled water. It is helpful to have various-sized funnels to limit the amount of spilling that will happen. And it will happen!

Dropper Bottles

Dropper bottles offer many uses. For the essential oil user, they can be especially valuable and offer another fantastic way to experience your oils.

Dropper bottles make using essential oils a lot simpler for larger applications. You can pre-blend your carrier oils and essential oils into a dropper bottle for use of facial serums, body oils, relaxation massage oils, dry skin serum, or to add to a bath. Droppers also allow for topical applications for larger surface areas.

Again, I use 4 oz. amber dropper bottles for any recipes. I simply fill the bottle ¾ of the way with carrier oil and add the oils needed for the recipe I am creating. Then I shake it up and start applying it. Dropper bottles make great gifts to share with friends and family!

My Daily Autoimmune Essential Oils

Although there are limited studies on the effect of essential oils for the autoimmune system, a few have demonstrated that they have a positive effect in easing various symptoms of my condition. Seriously, though, I don't pay attention to those studies. Who completed them anyway?

Since incorporating doTERRA oils into my health regimen, I

have noticed an improvement in both my physical and mental health. Oils provide me with something interesting to learn, research, and include into my daily life. We all need something fun to keep us busy.

Please remember, not all oils are created equal. So, when I talk about using oils internally, I'm specifically talking about doTERRA essential oils.

The primary essential oils that help me reduce inflammation, relieve pain, improve joint mobility, enhance relaxation, strengthen the bladder, lower anxiety, and create a sense of well-being are:

Frankincense

Warm and spicy frankincense is considered the "King of Oils." The uses and benefits are endless. Frankincense, when used internally, is able to stimulate the neurological system, increase the immune response, relieve anxiety, calm the mind, reduce inflammation, improve gut health, and more.

Topically, frankincense oil can help soothe and moisturize dry skin, promote a clear complexion, massage on abdomen to relieve cramps, and can help maintain healthy-looking fingernails. It also smells great mixed with lavender!

I even take 2 drops of frankincense internally (administered under my tongue) two times a day for three weeks, then take one week off and repeat the cycle. This way the oil gets absorbed directly into your GI tract and bloodstream.

Copaiba

The calming and woodsy aroma of copaiba is perfect for diffusing in your home. Copaiba works to protect the brain by interacting with the nervous system. It is known to be the most potent anti-inflammatory essential oil in the world.

When taken internally, copaiba can act as a powerful antioxidant to support a healthy immune system, protect the nervous system, and improve your mood while boosting joy and calming the mind.

Topically, due to copaiba's natural anti-inflammatory properties, it is a great essential oil to use for pain management and skin care.

I simply add a drop to a glass of water, 2 drops under my tongue, or use a roller bottle (dilute in a carrier oil) and apply to any sore areas that need some tender loving care. Every morning, I apply the roller to the soles of my feet, too!

Why the soles of my feet, you ask? The soles of the feet have much larger pores than the rest of our body. These pores are particularly absorbent and can quickly pull the essential oils into the bloodstream. This allows the benefits of the essential oils to reach multiple organs, systems, and areas of your body that are in need of support.

Helichrysum Oil

With the uplifting aroma of sweet fruit with honey, helichrysum is the perfect oil to use everywhere in the house. Referred to by some as the "Everlasting or Immortal Flower," the helichrysum plant offers several benefits to the skin, the neurological system, and can decrease muscle pain, reduce swelling and inflammation, and improve circulation.

Helichrysum essential oil has the ability to stimulate the neurological system to potentially ease various symptoms, including loss of balance, fatigue, impaired speech, bladder weakness, inflammation, and numbness or weakness of the limbs.

Topically, with a roller bottle, I apply the oil 2 times a day to my legs, soles of my feet, arms, wrists, back of the neck, and my temples. This oil has also worked wonders for my bladder, so I apply it on my lower stomach every morning and night. Adding basil and cypress oils can further enhance the circulation, decrease muscle tension, and reduce symptoms.

DAILY HOUSEHOLD USES

Nourishing Skin Care

What I enjoy most about applying essential oils with carrier oils for my own skin care is the fact that I make them myself with no chemicals or artificial ingredients, and it saves money. All natural, all the time!

USING AN AMBER DROPPER BOTTLE:
» Fill ¾ of the way with carrier oil
» Add 20 drops of essential oil (more or less depending on what you prefer): Lavender oil, rosehip oil, cypress oil, frankincense oil, peppermint oil, etc.
» Put lid on and shake, or roll in the palm of your hand

That's it! You have your very own DIY skin serum recipe. You can make as much or as little as you will need. I usually put a bottle in every bathroom instead of hand cream.

Essential Oil Sugar Scrub

Everyone loves a good exfoliating body scrub to polish the body, remove dead skin cells, and get glowing skin. Different sugars can be used to make a scrub like brown sugar, white sugar, or even raw sugar. It just depends on your preference.

USING A 4 OZ. MASON JAR ADD:
» ½ cup sugar
» ¼ cup fractionated coconut oil
» 6 drops lavender essential oil
» 6 drops citrus essential oil
» Mix all ingredients together in a bowl and place into the jar.

To use, scoop out a small amount and rub onto desired areas for exfoliating action.

Kitchen & Bathroom Counter Cleaner

This cleaning spray can be used in any room, providing a fresh, natural scent every time.

USING AN AMBER SPRAY BOTTLE ADD:
» 1 cup warm water
» 1 cup white vinegar
» 20 drops of a mix of essential oils: lavender, lemongrass, lemon, wild orange, peppermint, eucalyptus, on guard, purify, or tea tree

Bug Spray

This spray is used on the whole family, even the dog. I spray it on his collar before putting it on and then on his lower back (be careful to avoid the face and eyes).

USING AN AMBER SPRAY BOTTLE ADD:
» 1 cup distilled water
» ½ cup witch hazel
» 10 drops citronella
» 10 drops lemongrass
» 10 drops tea tree
» 5 drops lavender

LAUNDRY ROOM ESSENTIALS

Thanks to their deodorizing, antifungal, antibacterial, and cleaning properties, many essential oils work great for use in the laundry.

Fabric Softener

IN A 1L GLASS BOTTLE ADD
(or directly into washing machine cup):
» Fill bottle with white vinegar
» Add essential oils (20 drops for bottle or 3 drops into machine cup)
» Lavender for a calming and relaxing fragrance
» Citrus oil for deodorizing with a fresh scent
» Peppermint for an energizing boost
» Cinnamon for a warming and seasonal aroma
» Shake up the bottle to mix
» Fill washing machine cup

Wool Dryer Balls

» Add a couple of drops of your preferred essential oil to a dryer ball to keep the fragrance flowing.

5

Vitamins, Minerals & What!? Oh My!

Don't you always want to know what other people are doing to stay healthy? Aren't you curious about that athletic mom, or the wrinkle-free grandma who has more energy than you could ever dream of having? What do they do to stay healthy? Look around. Healthy people are everywhere. They look great, are full of oomph, and walk with a purpose (and not while holding a phone).

Now, I am not one of those women. I try, oh trust me, I try. Hair done, make-up on, breakfast eaten, kids lunches organized, beds made, dishes put away, exercise completed... Hold on; I just need to catch my breath.

To put it quite simply, some days are better than others. But no matter the day, I try to follow the same pattern when it comes to my vitamins/minerals/supplements/oils — basically stuff that I take every day.

But before we move on to my daily list, I want to take a moment to recommend checking with your healthcare practitioner before adding supplements to your diet. And always read and follow the directions on products.

SUCCESS #1: MORNING ACTIONS

Lemon Water

I use fresh lemons and squeeze the juice into my morning glass of water. Not only does it freshen your breath, it stimulates your digestive tract, provides Vitamin C, contains Potassium, and balances your body's pH levels. I only drink a few sips, but every little bit helps. NO Sugar!

St. Francis Herb Farm Strest Tincture

Basically I fill a shot glass with water (not very precise), add the drops, and consume in a single gulp. This helps regulate my stress while restoring my mental and emotional health and reducing any fatigue or anxiety. I don't consume this year-round, only when the stress of life takes over and I need additional support.

Fish Oil, MCT Oil, or FlaxSeed Oil

A spoonful of oil (makes the medicine go down, medicine go down...sing along) is enjoyed at breakfast. All oils are a concentrated source of Omega-3 fats (EPA and DHA) which benefit the heart, reduce inflammation, improve brain health, your mood, and the nervous system. I prefer the lemon flavored fish oil so there is no aftertaste or unwanted burps, and I add the MCT oil to my morning beverage or smoothie.

Vitamin D

A little drop of sunshine every day. Most people associate this with the sun and don't understand the full benefits it provides. Vitamin D is a nutrient that helps your body absorb calcium.

You can't have one without the other. Vitamin D helps you maintain healthy bones, increases energy, and protects against disease.

Multivitamin

I strive for balance in everything I do. I try to eat right, exercise more, and sleep better. But sometimes (okay, all the time), even when I am doing my best, life throws me a curve ball. In order to fill my nutrient gaps, I take a once-a-day multivitamin with breakfast.

Green Juice Powder and Collagen Powder

I mix these into my breakfast smoothie to get my added fruits, vegetables, greens, and additional health benefits for the day. I know what I (the whole family) should eat each day, but I also know what actually ends up being served at meal time. Of course I incorporate the various *Add-On, Add-In, Added To...* section items to it as well. (See page 113 for this list.)

Essential Oils (internally)

I take a drop of frankincense each morning and evening, a drop of DDR Prime with a turmeric capsule in the morning, and a drop of copaiba in the middle of the day. All drops are placed under my tongue (sublingual) in order to easily be absorbed through the thin mucous membranes there. This location allows the oil to bypass my digestion and become rapidly absorbed directly into the bloodstream. I use only doTERRA oils due to their purity and quality.

Essential Oils (topically)

I apply oils all day for various symptoms, support, and emotional healing. When getting dressed, I apply oils to my temples, neck, skull, wrists, soles of feet, abdomen, spine, and anywhere else that I can think of. The collection I have on my nightstand includes helichrysum, copaiba, cypress, lavender, rose, and adaptiv.

SUCCESS #2: EVENING ACTIONS

St. Francis Herb Farm Canadian Digestive Bitters

Before I sit down to eat, I use my shot glass again, add the required drops to water, and gulp. I take this to help with nutrient absorption, improve my digestion, and eliminate any potential gas or bloating.

Magnesium/Calcium

Magnesium has many benefits throughout all of the body's critical functions. This mineral supports healthy bones, nails, skin, hair, and teeth. It helps aid in restful sleep, relaxed muscles, and balances mood. The mineral calcium is important for optimal bone health throughout your life. The best way to get calcium is through your diet. If, however, you are like most people (or me), calcium supplements might be a good option.

Probiotics

Did you know that your immune system depends on the health of your gut (digestive tract)? Or that the digestive system is a large part of our neurological system? We really are what we eat. The entire family takes a probiotic with dinner.

Essential Oils

This is where my lavender roller bottle comes out. I basically lather myself, my pillow, my wrists, the soles of my feet, and then even rub my hands through my hair. The calming and relaxing aroma promotes a peaceful space, perfect for a restful sleep.

§

It seems like a lot of work, but keep it simple. Have everything handy and in a location that you can see. And if you forget, don't worry; there is always tomorrow.

HOW YOU DOIN'?

Talk about a loaded question! There are so many ways for this question to be asked. Let's explore.

How are you?
...asks your dear friend because she actually means it, and tilts her head while making eye contact.

How are you doing?
...asks a fellow co-worker who is just being polite.

How you doin'?
Could be a pick up line (think Joey from Friends), if said with an accent.

How are ya?
The quick and easy question with a jerk of the head as they pass you.

What's up?
Don't really care or even want to engage in any conversation.

How's it going? What's going on?
How have you been? How are you keeping?
Are you well?

The list goes on and on. Often it is a simple question that we misinterpret depending on our own personal mood that day. If we are happy and content with the world, it is a lovely question that we will joyfully answer. If we are down or tired, we might not even answer. Why bother? They don't really care anyway. Or if it was a quick head jerk, we get annoyed that anyone even acknowledged us in the first place.

It can be hard to respond when someone approaches me with this greeting. Do they honestly want to hear how I am feeling today? Should I share a personal thought or casually reply with my usual smile and say, "I'm fine. How are you?" Was the question genuine and from their heart? Would they be ready for the response I might offer where I honestly express all the feelings, emotions, and thoughts running around in my mind at that exact moment? Many times I don't want to share any information about myself, so my response is quick and to the point. I figure they don't fully understand what I go through day-to-day, so I keep the conversation basic and add in a bit of humour if I can.

Most people have good intentions and when someone takes the time to ask me, "How are you doing?" I recognize the effort it took on their part to ask. It can be frustrating navigating through life with an invisible illness.

I recognize that when someone sincerely wants to know how I am feeling, they will usually stop, focus on the moment, and take the time to listen to my response. I try to remember to do this for others as well. Everyone is dealing with life challenges in some way, whether it's an illness, family/work problems, or financial strain. So if I can be that person who takes the time to hear them, maybe someone will pay me back the same way.

Do you remember that movie with the concept of paying it forward? Well, I try to include this in my daily life. I believe that the universe has my back, and that what goes around comes around. So if I do something meaningful for another human being, I will see it come back to me in unexpected ways. Here's my favourite example: I usually use a coupon for the movie theatre and often forget that the concession snack comes with a regular popcorn and two drinks. So because I love (LOVE) popcorn, I order another bag of popcorn (for myself, the regular size is not enough to share!) with a drink. Now, I have three drink cups to fill and only two adults are attending the movie.

So I pass the empty cup to the person behind me in line, that way they don't need to order a drink. That's a decent-sized savings for a family of four, with everyone ordering popcorn and a drink. Anything free is helpful. I love the surprise and joy that it brings people. It is such an effortless act of kindness.

One year it was repaid to me with a turkey! I'll keep the story short. At the grocery store, the lady in front of me acquired a free turkey due to the store promotion but didn't want it (What? It's Thanksgiving this weekend!). So she asked me if I would like it. Hell yes! Then I thanked her and the universe for this free turkey.

So don't overthink a friendly greeting or gesture. Start a conversation and be social. And if it was a pick up line, good for you! You've still got it.

6

Just Move it, Move it!

So you have an illness and you want to feel better? Or do you want to build muscle? Some days, all you want to do is curl into a ball and hide away, especially in snowy or rainy weather. Exercise is an important part of your health and treatment plan. Exercise can actually strengthen your mind, reduce inflammation, improve your mood, and reduce fatigue. Plus, physical activity has been shown to increase your endurance, muscle strength, and brain health.

Finding the time to exercise and getting motivated to even get started — whether you have an illness or not — is hard. I can come up with excuses every day to delay the process: work, write, tidy up, put dishes away, bake cookies, take the dog for a walk, read, etc. And trust me, I usually do! But when I finally push myself to begin my daily practice, I feel great afterwards.

MOTION IS LOTION

No matter how small it might seem, put your body in motion every day. Stretch your arms to the sky, roll your shoulders, move your head up and down, stretch to the side, shake your hips, touch (or try to touch) your toes, point and flex your feet, lunge from side-to-side, walk around your house, lay on your back, hug your knees, and *breathe*. Small movements each day will bring lubrication into your weary bones. More motion equals more blood flow, and your spirit will be lifted.

My exercises revolve around five key areas: stretching, aerobic movement, strength/resistance training, functional mobility, and meditation.

1) Stretching

I always stretch and do light movements to start off my exercise sessions. This helps me maintain my range of motion. They are pretty boring, actually. I start in a standing position or seated, begin my joint mobility routine, and end up stretching on the carpet. This entire section takes about ten to fifteen minutes to complete, moving from my head all the way to my feet with five reps each.

- » **Start by moving your head to the left & right, up & down, side to side, and front to back.**

- » **Rotate your shoulders backward, forward, then shrug them up and down.**

- » **Roll your elbows inward and outward.**

- » **Rotate your wrists, flap your hands up and down, and do wrist waves (clasping your hands together).**

- » **Move your fingers, bend, stretch, and play air piano.**

- » **Move and shake your hips in all directions.**

- » **Swing each leg frontward/backward and then side to side. (Sometimes I stand on the bottom stair to help my left leg move better.)**

» **For the knees, kick each leg in and out, side to side, and in circles. (Again, I use the stairs.)**

» **Point and flex the ankles and rotate in circles. Sit if you have to and rotate with your hands.**

» **Toes can be squeezed, released, and pressed into the ground.**

I will then stretch my arms up to the ceiling and bend forward to touch the ground or the back of a chair a few times before sitting on the carpet.

» **I start with frog stretch (soles of feet together, knees bent) and bend forward to feet and side to side to each knee.**

» **Lift right arm up and stretch the right side of the body.**

» **Lift left arm up and stretch the left side of the body.**

» **Straighten out one leg, head to knee.**

» **Straighten out other leg, head to knee.**

» **Straighten both legs, try to touch feet.**

» **Lay down and hug both knees.**

» **Stretch right leg out, hug left knee.**

» **Switch and stretch left leg out, hug right knee.**

» **Sit up and move onto all fours.**

» **Cat and dog stretch.**

2) Aerobic Movement

Aerobic exercise is so important as it increases your heart rate and blood flow. The problem for me is how to get it. With any lack of mobility, use of aids, and overall fatigue, this component is hard most days. I like to accomplish everything in small batches. A bit here and there goes a long way!

Be creative. What are some activities you enjoy that incorporate movement? I like:

» **Dance (standing or sitting) for an entire song or two. Swing your arms if that is what works best for you.**

» **While standing, pump your arms, kinda like punching, to the front, side, and above your head.**

» **Walk inside or outside your house, counting your steps.**

» **Go to the store and do a few laps in the aisles (while pushing the cart).**

» **Complete housework.**

» **While cooking, move around, swing your arms, march in place, and just keep moving.**

3) Strength/Resistance

It is important to maintain and improve your body's muscle strength. With the use of free weights, machines, bands, and household items, you can do this anywhere. Keep the weight at a reasonable amount, do repetitions, and work the muscles throughout your body.

Here is my program:

» **2-lb. hand weights or with resistance bands: 2 sets of 10 — bicep curl, chest press, overhead shoulder press, straight arm front lift, and straight arm side lift.**

» **Modified Stair/Wall Push Ups: 2 sets of 10 — with seated hip stretches between sets. I like the pigeon pose. Sitting upright on the stairs, cross your right ankle over your left knee and bend forward. Then switch sides. This is also where I complete ankle rotations.**

4) Functional Mobility

Functional movements are exercises that engage multiple muscle groups at the same time. Think of them as functions that you do each day, like getting out of bed, getting up and down from a chair, in and out of the car, or lifting groceries. These can be very helpful because they train the muscles to continue performing daily tasks effectively and safely. You can perform functional movements with or without weights, and they can be incorporated into a strength/resistance routine easily (most strength moves are, in fact, functional movements).

Effective movement depends on how your brain and nerves communicate with your muscles and joints in the body. This will translate into increased coordination, balance, and flexibility for you. Some of the functional exercises I perform are:

» **Chair routine: 2 sets of 10 — sit to stand position (chair squat), knee lifts, knee extensions, tummy twist, and calf raises.**

» **Stair routine: 2 sets of 10 — stair climbs (take a**

controlled step up with the right foot and slowly step back down; repeat with left leg)

» **Walk as much as you can — concentrate on proper walking: swinging your arms, lifting your legs, and placing your heel down. This is more difficult for my left leg, so I take it slowly.**

5) Meditation

First, a bit about meditation. I have always wanted to meditate. The cool, calm people do it! But I used to think it was hard. I could not sit and concentrate on breathing while emptying my thoughts. Come on! I am a woman and my brain is in multitask mode most of the time, so even the thought of meditating made me cringe.

Meditation plays a key role in my exercise program now, though. I like to end my routine with this practice so that I can give thanks to my body for allowing me to complete my exercises, take a breath, and get centered for the rest of my day.

Meditation can be done anywhere and anytime. There are numerous resources to help guide and teach you. The internet is a wonderful resource. There are guided versions on YouTube, inspirational websites, and even apps you can use on your phone or tablet.

Meditation is a tool that can be forgotten or put off in a flash. Making it a habit will change your life. Some of the benefits that I have experienced from a regular meditation routine are:

» **Allows me to recharge so that I have more energy throughout the day.**

» **Clears my mind and increases my focus.**

» **Attracts quiet into my morning. A sense of peace and tranquility.**

Needless to say, there are a ton of benefits of adopting a regular meditation practice, and these are just a few of them that I have noticed.

§

All of these exercise ideas can be completed at home, in a gym, or with a physical therapist. Be careful. Have all of the necessary tools that you might need (e.g. I like having the couch or a bed beside me, to help me brace myself if needed). Play some music, stay cool, and make it a fun experience for yourself.

7

Virus in the House

Virus in the house! I REPEAT... VIRUS IN THE HOUSE! Alert, Alert...Wee-oh wee-oh wee-oh (fire truck sound)

Too dramatic? All I'm saying is that a virus — whether a stuffy nose, tummy ache, headache, or fever — has entered the building. The thought of anyone getting sick often sends parents into overdrive. They stop thinking, start looking up information on the internet, grab the first medicine bottle they can find, and usually just overreact in general.

It can be really hard to stay calm when your child (especially a baby) shows symptoms of a cold. Having an autoimmune illness does not help this situation, as no one wants me to get sick and possibly bring on a flare-up. We are not doctors; we only have our common sense, knowledge, memories of what our parents did, or what we have heard that needs to be done.

So I am telling you this: I've been there and done that. My advice is to slow down, breathe, and start asking yourself logical questions. If it is your baby, ask your trusted circle of family and friends what they think. I do advise that you consult with your doctor if the symptoms are unique, different from the seasonal variety, or new to you.

My kids are healthy most of the time, but they do get the seasonal cold. It has taken me years to feel confident and trust myself to do the right thing. I have a pattern that I follow, and over the years, various friends have asked me for ideas. So I thought the best way to share them would be to put it into my book.

You see, I don't follow all of the traditional medical protocols. As you can probably tell from my section titled *Alternative Medicine: My Journey Into the Unknown*, incorporating various complementary medicines — to ease the symptoms for everyone in the house before I rush out to the germ-infested doctor's office and wait to see a professional — is my plan.

Okay, let's start to tackle this bug!

1) Ask questions to whomever the patient might be (if a baby, then ask yourself). How do they feel? What is bothering them the most? When did they first notice this? Sometimes this is easy, as you heard the cough or you can tell they have a fever just by looking at them.

2) Record when the symptoms started and what they were (keep a journal). Morning time, during the day at school, at dinner, or during the night?

3) Engage them to talk (if they are old enough). Listen to their voice. Look at their eyes. Are they red or puffy? Follow their gestures. Are they standing, sitting, holding their head, or hugging a Kleenex box? Do they sound tired, normal, angry, or anxious? Did they lay down immediately? Did they go straight to bed in a dark room and cover their head with the sheets?

4) Feel for heat. If they have a fever, is their forehead warm? Usually their eyes are glossy, red, and irritated. Check their body/chest for warmth. How about their hands and feet — are they warm or cold?

5) Look at the mucus (I know, gross) or ask them, "Is your nose running or is it congested?" Is the mucus watery or thick? Can they blow their nose or is it already dripping on its own? This gets easier as they get older; they will tell you before you even ask.

6) If it is vomiting or a stomach ache, I put them into bed, usually with a large plastic bowl beside them and a glass of water, or sit them in front of the toilet. Now all we do is wait for everything to come out. No use putting anything else into their delicate bodies. Get that virus out!

Once I gather all of my information, I can start to think and research (from my journal or books) what to do to help ease any pain. This is why I encourage keeping a journal, so you can refer back to what treatments you followed last time. The immune system has to be able to do its job, so I want to create an environment to encourage it to do so.

At this point I will dive into my remedy chest — (that sounds so authentic!) — which is just the kitchen cupboard that houses most of our paraphernalia to deal with the immune system.

MY ESSENTIALS

Drink

Start by getting lots of liquids into the diet. I like warm honey lemon water, warm lemon ginger bone broth, and soups.

Sleep

A good night's sleep is essential for good health. When you sleep, your body begins to repair itself and healing begins.

Wet Socks

This approach feels nasty but it works. Before going to bed, soak a pair of socks in cold water. Then wring them out and immediately place them on the feet (ooh!). Now cover the wet socks with a dry pair of socks. This approach triggers a response from the body that relieves nasal congestion and prompts the body to increase circulation, which speeds up the activity of your immune system. Follow the steps for a few nights, and notice how sleep has improved. It sounds weird and unbelievable but it really does work.

Chiropractor

This is the first doctor that we visit if we need to see someone. The adjustment will loosen congestion and increase immune system activity for faster recovery.

Colloidal Silver

This tasteless water provides immune support and antibacterial benefits for a variety of symptoms. For a sore throat or a cough, gargle with a spoonful.

Bee Propolis Throat Spray

Propolis is a fast-acting, germ-fighting spray that contains numerous beneficial vitamins and minerals. It soothes and relieves coughs and sore throats.

Vitamin D

An important vitamin that helps your muscles, nerves, and immune system to work properly. A drop or two in the morning can help to battle the virus.

Probiotics

A valuable tool to use during any illness. They can enhance your immune function, helping to fight the common cold. Follow the directions on the label and start to combat the symptoms.

Homeopathy Remedies

A natural approach to wellness. Over time, I have acquired basic remedies to work for common illnesses that pop up. While our first instinct (especially as parents) may be to purchase over-the-counter medication to resolve complaints, there are often natural remedies that don't interfere with the body's own immune system and can help ease uncomfortable symptoms.

There are also some great pre-packaged homeopathic remedies from your pharmacy that are marketed for teething, flu or cough symptoms. Learning a little homeopathy can go a long way to ease your mind and nervous system when dealing with a virus.

Note: I am not a doctor, so this section is for informational purposes only and is not intended to be used as a replacement when medical attention is required.

I CAN. I WILL.
Watch Me.

*O*nce diagnosed, like it or not, your life has changed. You tell yourself that most people will face a devastating diagnosis at some point in their life. It might be a personal illness, a child's sickness, or an elderly parent's chronic symptoms. You tell yourself anything to keep a grip on your emotions, even finding ways to be grateful on a daily basis.

One of the soul-crushing challenges of dealing with any medical conclusion is that you have no idea how it will affect you. You might suffer immediate symptoms. Others can be prolonged with intervention, or nothing really manifests for years. The uncertainty is just as bad as the diagnosis itself.

The initial shock can be overwhelming, confusing, or may not make any sense at all. As for myself, I did not know anything about MS. In the beginning years, I looked to the medical community to treat my symptoms. Wake up, I feel good, so I go about my day. Wake up, I feel bad...so I book a doctor's appointment so they can make me feel better. It was the usual cycle of feeling crappy and grabbing the medicine. I would feel better for a while, then feel bad again, triggering another doctor's visit. I hated it.

Over the years I found ways to prepare myself for my challenging future. I welcomed a new medical team that includes natural practitioners. I still see my neurologist once a year, but I try not to listen to negative feedback. Doctors, in all their wisdom, can be real downers. It is their job to prepare us, even educate us, on what the future might hold, but I seriously don't want to be told that my legs are going to start getting weaker. Thanks, now that thought is in my head and I am starting to believe it! CRAP.

MY 5-STEP PROCESS

1) Build a Support Team

This can be a team of people that you meet with, it can be your family, people you follow on social media, meet at events, or even just watch on TV. I prefer to do my research, align all my medical and holistic practitioners that I feel inspired by, and spread information on healthy living with my family.

2) Ask for Help

Being a Taurus, this is a hard one for me. As the chapter title sums it up perfectly, *I CAN. I WILL. WATCH ME.* My challenge is to allow others to help me, and their challenge is to find a way that does not overwhelm or intrude on my space. Learning how to ask for help is the big one for me. I remind myself that most people like to help and usually feel relieved to have a chance to make your life a bit more manageable.

3) Take Control of Your Health

Read that again. *TAKE CONTROL OF YOUR HEALTH.*

Only you have control of your body, mind, and spirit. You determine how you will feel today and what you can accomplish. The medical world can provide you with all the information about your condition, but you have to take control of your health and how you respond to the life-altering diagnosis you've been handed.

4) Gather Information for Your Future

Read, read, and read some more. Gather information about how you want to live, how you want to feel, and how you want to thrive. Become educated on the illness and then start living. I don't really like to read about medical research or even that much about my illness. I personally don't find it encouraging, unless it is a new, well-tested approach. So thank you for reading my book if you have an autoimmune illness.

I do like to read success stories and be inspired by people. Exploring various therapies that have helped others, alternative strategies to supplement my current care, and embracing a healthy lifestyle are what motivate me.

5) Find Ways to Live With Uncertainty

The bad news is that no matter how much treatment I undergo, how many healthy lifestyle changes I make, or how much support I have, I cannot change the uncertainty of my illness. No two days are ever the same. My goal is to find ways to help slow the illness down or find the best way to learn how to deal with it.

Many people begin their healing journey feeling confused and overwhelmed. Then devastation creeps in when that new exercise plan or miracle drug fails to cure the illness. Ultimately, you must find empowering ways to cope, thrive, survive, and even shine in this new chapter of your life.

The right strategy varies for everyone. Set up a daily routine, a meal guide, an exercise program, a monthly calendar, basically a new life plan. This can actually bring creativity and direction to your days. So have fun and go live your life to the fullest.

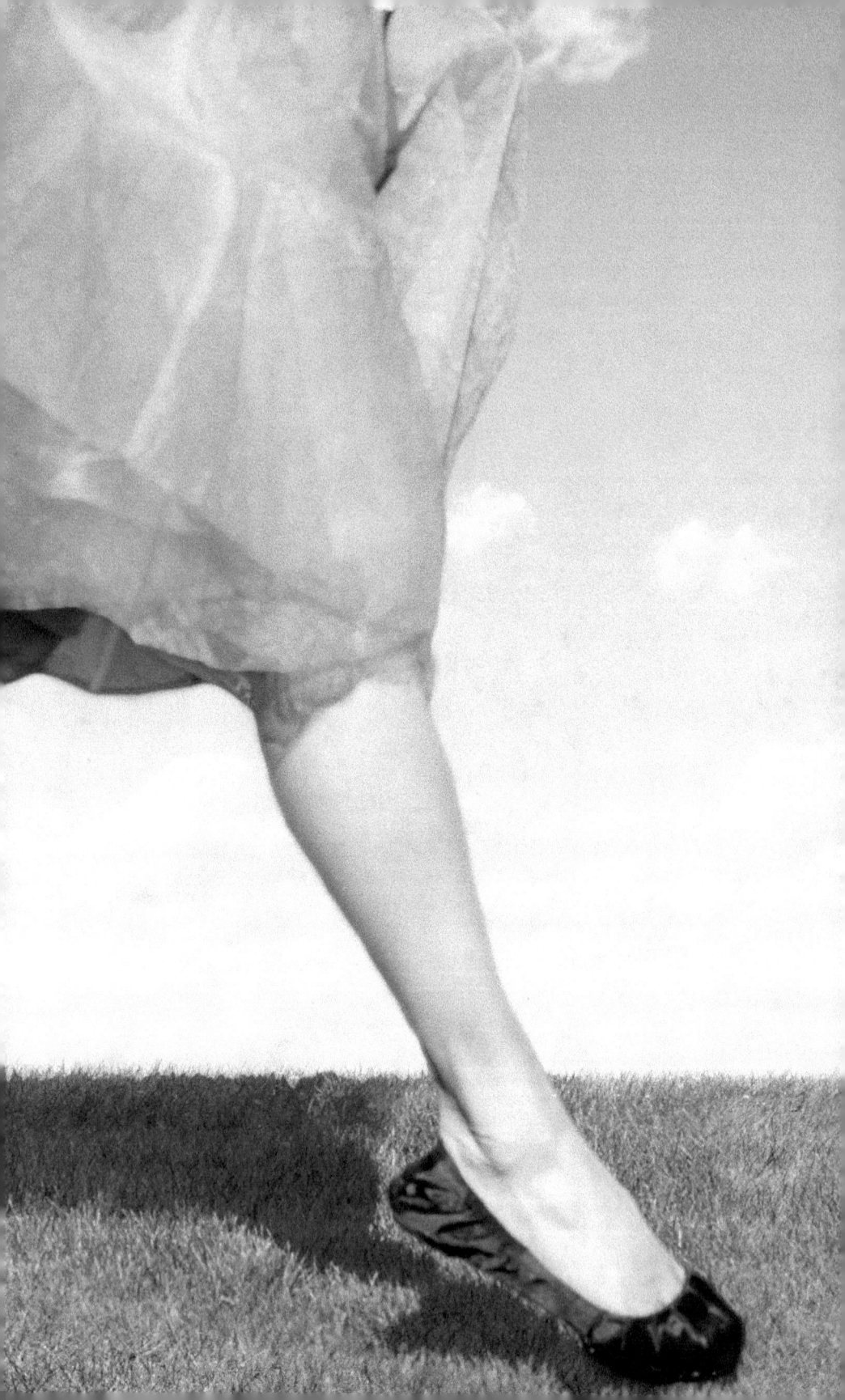

Part Three

PERSONAL CARE

8

Self-Care

*T*he quality of your life is up to you. You get to decide who and what affects you. The world is full of information that can break you down or lift you up. It is your job to protect yourself and flourish in your life.

It is important to remember that it is not what you say to anybody else or what they say to you that matters; it is the conversation that you have with yourself every day. Being grateful and kind to anyone who crosses your path — including yourself — is vital to your mental state.

Each morning, I remind myself that it will be a great day. I also remind myself of these five uplifting points to move forward in my journey on a daily basis:

1) I don't need other people's permission to be myself. I am "good enough" and I accept myself enough to make every day fabulous.

2) When I am having a bad day, I make sure to be extra kind to myself. I allow myself to find a way to feel better and surround myself with positive thoughts.

3)   I don't allow my thoughts to center on other people's opinions. My personal expectations of success and happiness for me might be completely different from others.

4)   Notice ways to be positive. Your ultimate defense against stress is to choose to be happy and think empowering thoughts. You have to reduce the outside negative noise.

5)   The daily quality of your life depends upon how you set and respect your priorities for the day. It's not selfish to love yourself, take care of yourself, and do what is right for you. So if staying home and sitting on the couch is what you need, then go for it.

DAILY TO-DO: SELF-CARE

Be gentle with yourself. Stop comparing yourself to anyone, anywhere, ever! We all feel the pressure to improve our lives, whether financially, nutritionally, physically, or spiritually. Stop holding yourself to a standard that you have viewed on social media. Guess what? That crap has been edited, retouched, rehearsed, and scheduled. You are the boss of your life, your health, and your well-being.

The best place to start self-care is in finding the simplicity of day-to-day tasks. Taking small steps on a continuous basis will add up to big changes over the year. Trying to make gigantic changes too fast will overwhelm you. Life is already fully packed with work, cooking, cleaning, kids, parents, pets, exercising — so start the simplification process slowly.

As a woman and a perfectionist (at times), I get in my own way. Learn to relax. You don't need to see the benefits 100% for them to work. The results will come, and if you are centered in your body and soul, the results can be celebrated: love, peace, joy, and gratitude.

With self-care on your mind, try to complete just one item listed below on a daily basis:

» **Start your day with introspection, stretches, and affirmations.**

» **Nourish your body. Drink water and eat your fruits and veggies.**

» **Take charge of your health. Book that appointment, try a new therapy, and become intentionally involved in your health care.**

» **Go outside: sit in the sun, breathe in the fresh air, and play with the dog — anything that grounds you.**

» **Indulge in a real conversation, not by text. Reach out and call someone. Answer a text by calling them. They will be pleasantly surprised.**

» **Be present. Don't be distracted or try to multitask. Concentrate on what is happening around you, within you, and observe the moment.**

Learn to take your self-care seriously.

You are worth every minute that you spend on yourself. Take the time to rest, replenish, restore, and revive. You have the power, and luckily, are in charge of your life. NOW GO!

9

Meal Planning, Batch Cooking, or Pantry Party?

This is something that I struggle with. I don't enjoy cooking (or even food much, for that matter). It is a constant learning curve for me, and it starts with the dreaded breakfast: eggs (again), bagel with cream cheese, or cereal with berries.

When I was first navigating how to live with my newfound illness, I met again with that chiropractor who first adjusted me for my supposed pinched nerve. He stressed the important role that nutrition plays and shared his nutritional sciences degree knowledge on this subject.

He did not charge me for this or prescribe anything to me. We just talked. He talked about the history of farming, changes in production practices over the years, vitamins and nutrients, and the importance of each meal. He discussed the role that marketing plays in the consumption of food, the dangers of processed foods, and to think about enjoying the simple ingredients found in basic food.

I remember walking away with one specific tidbit of knowledge that I have followed and still stick to each day: start your day with protein! It is the best way to fuel your body for the day.

So I started having shakes or smoothies every single morning. Protein, fruit, greens, omega oils, seeds, nut butter, and anything healthy is added to the blender. Every few days I mix up two jars so that in the mornings I can just reach into the fridge, shake it up, and pour a glass.

I try to take a step back and make an actual effort to end all of the mealtime madness. It is easier than you think, so stop overthinking it. You'll get frustrated. Trust me, I did at first. So I have simplified it into five steps. Take a deep breath and read on.

Picture this: you just got home from work or from picking up the kids. Everyone is hungry and you all run into the kitchen to grab a cookie. Nothing has been planned for dinner. You open the fridge/freezer/pantry, but nothing is satisfying your desire to cook. So frozen pizza/lasagna or take out it is...but you'll add some cut up vegetables on the table to increase the nutritional value.

You plan your daily work, kids activities, and exercise schedule, but do you really (be honest) think out what you are going to eat each day? And who knew that becoming an adult would involve so much cooking? We have to eat with a purpose to nourish and fuel our bodies. It sounds easy, but with our crazy, overworked, over-scheduled, over-interrupted lives, we often forget or just push it aside all together. Then Monday comes again and we are right back to our crazy schedule and the need to grocery shop.

In this section, I'll lead you through my simple 5-step process and show you my weekly plan. When you begin to think about meals ahead of time, create shopping lists, and cook with the future in mind, working in the kitchen will become fun again (kind of).

If you're the boss in the kitchen, you'll feel healthier mentally and physically. This is something that I have always had a hard time with, as cooking is not something that I truly enjoy. But if I can be creative, create a colorful meal strategy plan to follow, and work from a list, I'm in a happy place.

The internet is a wealth of information on this matter, with numerous ideas, guides, and apps to help you along. I choose to keep my life uncomplicated. I rarely do a big Sunday meal prep routine. I just can't find the time to complete this with only two hands. Between the laundry, homework, dog, cleaning, and family fun, the day flies by. I will, however, work on chopping and cooking some veggies, washing lettuce, cutting up fruit, and I always accomplish some baking (muffins, cookies, snack bars) for the weekday school lunches.

All of our meals are prepared in large batches. This can start on Saturday morning with breakfast pancakes, waffles, French toast, eggs and bacon. We make double recipes and keep the additional items in the fridge for weekday mornings. Bacon is perfect for sandwiches, added to salads, or for a quick after school snack. My husband is great at weekend meals, so we always BBQ various meats and prepare a huge pot of chili or a roast.

FOLLOW MY FABULOUS 5

Fab 1 — Calendar Time

Take out your calendar and identify the days that you need quick meals. Think about lunches. When do you personally need to pack a lunch? What days do you have meetings? Will you be in the office or traveling around? What nights do you have appointments, social events, or kids' activities?

Fab 2 — Take Inventory

Get out a piece of paper and a pen. Now start writing down all of the food that you have in stock. Make note of anything that needs to be consumed ASAP (look at the expiration dates if you have to). Notice the basics: the vegetables, the frozen items, meats, beverages, and even the baked goods. Start getting ideas of what you can cook.

Fab 3 — Meals

Label the type of meals you will need each day and night. It could be a meal that you have to cook from scratch, a meal that is prepped (frozen) and ready to go into the oven, a fully cooked meal that just needs reheating, or a simple side dish to add to the delicious dinner that has been in the slow cooker all day.

This is the stage where I will start to get ideas. Get out those cookbooks, websites, or hand-written notes and pick some of your favorite recipes.

» Remember to pick a protein for every meal. We usually rotate between chicken, beef, veggie beef, seafood, and eggs. If you are a vegetarian, then do the same thing with veggie protein options.

» Pick recipes with lots of healthy choices. Add salads, vegetables and dips.

» Use lots of colors.

Fab 4 — Choose the Meal

Fill in your calendar (or a separate meal planning page) with the meal you will be serving each day. Include the side dishes needed. Here's an example — Monday: BBQ Chicken with oven roasted vegetables and Greek salad. Hint: I pick up a BBQ chicken so all I have to do is take out the pre-cut vegetables from the fridge (or freezer), put them in the oven with the chicken, and toss the salad. Then, usually, your lunch section gets filled in automatically based on your previous evening's dinner.

Fab 5 — Grocery List Time

Your meal planning is complete, the meals are entered into the days, and you can now create the shopping list. Keep your inventory list handy and add the missing ingredients. I prefer to create the list in the order that they appear in the store to expedite the shopping experience even more! My list goes in order of: produce, bakery, meat, fish, dairy, frozen, and then packaged goods. When it comes to actual shopping, I choose to walk around the perimeter before I venture into the aisles. Or, better yet, if I am really planning ahead, I purchase all fresh foods from the local market and order packaged goods online for delivery or pick-up. I prefer to order meat online and have enough to fill the basement freezer for a few months

When it comes to shopping, I like to do it in bulk. I will purchase two or three of everything (especially if it is on sale). That way I can cook in large quantities. A perfect example is the BBQ chicken. I purchase two; one to be used for dinner and the other to be stored in the freezer. Having two growing teenagers in the house does not leave many leftovers, but if I cook double the portion sizes, I am usually left with extra to pack for lunches or leftovers for another day.

There you go. You are done. That is my easy-peasy, anyone-can-do-it Fabulous Five. The name just sounds fun! Go ahead now and enjoy your food.

FABULOUS EXTRA THOUGHT: GIVE THANKS AND ENJOY YOUR FAMILY

Be mindful when you are eating that delicious meal you just whipped up for everyone. This is a great time to get the kids in the kitchen with no distractions. Have them set the table, prep or cook with you, fill the drink cups, and serve the plates (they also clear the table afterward and do the dishes).

Be present in the moment, aware of what is on your plate, learning about everyone's day, sharing stories, and enjoying the simple task of eating delicious food. Make dinner fun again!

LEST WE FORGET:
THE DREADED SCHOOL LUNCH

School lunches seem to be an enormous headache for most parents. The thought of what to pack, the time spent preparing, and then time spent unpacking at the end of the day can be so aggravating. Usually, it seems like nothing was eaten. All containers come home just as they left in the morning: full of food. (Rest assured, this does change as they become teenagers!)

I tend to streamline this daily task and break it down to **5 Fabulous** requirements for what to pack everyday:

Fab 1) Fruit: grapes, pineapple, oranges, apples, etc.

Fab 2) Treat: cookies, brownies, muffins
(Sunday baking put to use).

Fab 3) Vegetables: carrots, cucumbers, pickles, tomatoes, etc.

Fab 4) Main item: sandwich, leftovers, soup, salad, chicken, stew, etc.

Fab 5) Drink: bottle of water.

I really only have to worry about the main item component each day, as the fruit and veggies are cut up and ready to go in the fridge and the treats are in the cookie jar. As long as everyone has healthy food choices, my job is done. Now if only they would eat everything!

JUST RUNNING OUT TO THE STORE!

*S*ometimes I forget that I have MS. I want to move. I want to shop. I want to do everything, get it done, and fast. Here is a breakdown of how I run out to the store to quickly grab the essentials.

I wake up, stretch before getting out of bed, and carefully make my way downstairs to the kitchen. Then I make my protein breakfast shake, sit down and drink it all, slowly climb upstairs to get dressed, put my makeup on, do my hair, concentrate on descending the stairs to the main level, let the dog out, bring the dog back in, go to the bathroom, get my phone, check emails/texts/calls, confirm the weather, pack my purse, go to the bathroom (my shake was a lot of liquid), sit down to put on my shoes and ankle brace, find my cane, and slowly make my way out the door. I walk to the car, using the side of the house as a stabilizer until I reach the driver's side door, drop my cane into the passenger side, and gently lower myself into the driver's seat. Then I sit in the car for a few minutes to recover from the exhaustion of the morning so far. I am finally ready to drive off.

Once at the store, I park near the carts because they are easier to walk with than a cane. (Which reminds me! Why are all of the cart parking sections so far away from the handicap parking?!) I make my way into the store, take out my shopping list, and start on my slow trek through the aisles (and it is slow). My trips are not swift shopping visits. Running out to grab something doesn't happen in my life anymore. It can be a 2 hour-long adventure, but that is okay with me. I take my time and pace myself. I fill my cart, looking for sale items while always checking my list so that I don't return home missing an important ingredient for dinner. I tend to finish up by using the bathroom — yes, again. Then I find a small cashier line and wait my turn. I chat with anyone in front of or behind me — the cashier, the impatient shopper, or the mom with the adorable baby. Almost done! Time to bag up the groceries and make my way back to my parked car.

Taking my time (even though another car has decided to stop and wait for my spot), I arrange all of the bags in the trunk. I spread out the heavy ones, the frozen items, the packaged products, the lightweight goodies, and the large boxes. Everything is a structured plan for my return home. What needs to be brought into the house immediately? What bags can wait until after school for my kids to carry into the house? Then I take the cart back to its area and walk (with my cane) to my car that is parked too far away. All the while, the intrusive car is still waiting and watching my every move.

Whew, getting tired folks! Actually, I'm completely worn out. The drive home will be useful to rest my weary legs.

Shopping done, check! Now a whole new adventure awaits: arriving back at home and unpacking the car. I won't go into too much detail, but you can imagine this takes me multiple trips just to unload a few bags with the use of only one hand. All necessary bags are placed in the kitchen, perishable food put away in the fridge or freezer, dog let out, dog let back in, glass of water poured, phone in hand, and I make my way to the computer to check on any business emails.

This is my full morning. It usually takes about three hours to fully complete the grocery shopping from start to finish.

My energy is completely drained and I have to rest my legs and try to get some strength back. I will not move for a good twenty minutes.

I forgot I have MS. I don't really forget. I just think that I can do everything the same way I used to. But I did way too much. My body/mind/spirit is weary.

But I can do it. I want to do it, and I will do it. I have learned to plan and pay a price for living a normal life (what looks "normal" to those watching).

So I plan. All of the details are thought out, timing considerations taken, driving routes mapped, and bathroom locations confirmed. My family is used to it and I am used to it. It has become my way of life. It's funny how quickly we can adapt to a new way of doing things. I am just thankful that I can accomplish what I need to. I might be slower, but I am still moving.

10

Add-On, Add-In, Added To... You Get My Point

*E*ating the right foods at every meal, watching how much of certain ingredients I have consumed, and trying to remember what I just ate yesterday can be daunting (for me, at least)! So I try to incorporate some extra nutrition on every plate by increasing my "Add-on," "Add-in," and "Added to" items in daily dishes. I do this for every member of the family...even the dog!

Here are my favorite nourishing additions:

CHIA SEEDS — STRONG LIKE BULL

Are you eating chia seeds? Have you heard of them? Chia seeds are little black seeds that are a nutrient-dense and energy-boosting superfood to have in the kitchen.

Chia Seeds Contain:

» Calcium
» Iron
» Potassium
» Protein

» Antioxidants
» Magnesium
» Omega 3

Chia Seed Benefits:

1) **Skin and aging**
   Chia seeds are one of nature's highest antioxidant foods.

2) **Digestive health**
   Chia seeds are very high in fiber.

3) **Heart health**
   Chia seeds have the ability to reverse inflammation, regulate cholesterol, and lower blood pressure.

4) **Boosts your energy**
   Chia seeds provide you with stable energy due to the ratio of protein, fat, and fiber.

5) **Stronger bones**
   Chia seeds contain calcium. Just 1 ounce has about 18 percent of the recommended daily amount.

Enjoy Chia Seeds by Adding Them to:

» **Smoothies & green juices**
» **Make chia seed pudding**
» **Muffins and baked goods**

Great Egg Recipe Alternative: Substitute one egg with 1 tablespoon chia seeds and let soak in 1/3 cup water for 15 minutes. The gel-like consistency creates the same binding quality that eggs possess.

HEMP HEARTS — SUPERFOOD TO THE RESCUE!

Hemp hearts are the shelled seeds of the hemp plant. They are tiny seeds with a very, very subtle nutty taste. They are known to have the most concentrated amount of protein, essential fatty acids, and vitamins around. I have been incorporating hemp hearts regularly for years, pretty much at every meal.

Hemp Hearts Contain:

» **Protein**
» **Fibre**
» **Iron**
» **Calcium**
» **Vitamin A, B2, B6, B1, C, D3 & E**

Benefits of Hemp Hearts (in a nutshell):

1) **Packed with protein**
   Hemp is a complete protein containing amino acids.
   Protein is so important in our diet as it is responsible
   for making neurotransmitters — the internal messaging
   system that sends signals throughout your body to make it
   work properly.

2) **High in fibre**
   Fibre is important for digestive health, keeps blood sugar
   levels stable, and is great for weight maintenance.

3) **Perfect balance of omega essential fats**

4) **They are antioxidant-rich**
   Full of vitamins, hemp hearts are bursting with
   antioxidants that can neutralize dangerous free radicals
   and contribute to overall health.

5) **Full of essential minerals**
   Inside these little seeds you will find potassium, zinc,
   calcium, magnesium and iron.

Enjoy Hemp Hearts

The options are endless when it comes to adding hemp hearts to your diet. As they are full of protein, I tend to sprinkle them on everyone's breakfast.

» **Sprinkle on toast with peanut butter, honey, or jam**
» **On cooked vegetables**
» **Oatmeal or cereal**
» **Muffins and baked goods**
» **Hummus & guacamole dips**

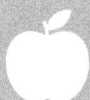

I would suggest storing hemp hearts (as well as chia seeds) in the refrigerator. Seeds contain precious oils that can spoil quickly.

COLLAGEN POWDER — YOUR SECRET WEAPON!

Yes, collagen! You know it from your body lotions, face creams, and even hair products. But did you know that collagen is found in our muscles, skin, bones, digestive system, joints, and even our gums inside the mouth? It is one of the largest proteins in our body. And, kids need collagen, too! It is the protein that our human bodies need as we age. As a mother of two very busy, athletic, clever children, I am very conscious of what my kids eat, drink, and consume each day.

Collagen Contains:

» **Amino acids**
» **Protein**

The great thing about this powder is that it is tasteless and odorless. It's a perfect trick for moms to use and add to meals without the kids even knowing.

Some Benefits of Collagen:

1) **Improves health of skin**

   As you read this, your collagen production is declining. Don't worry, it happens naturally to everyone. Increasing your collagen can help firm up, increase smoothness, and improve the elasticity of your skin.

2) **Reduces joint pain and repairs connective tissue**

   Do you ever wake up feeling stiff and slow to move in the morning? I tend to blame it on my illness, but that isn't always the case. My sore muscles and overworked tendons & ligaments need some love from the inside by consuming collagen.

3) **Calms anxiety**

   Collagen contains amino acids that have the ability to calm and balance various moods.

4) **Helps leaky gut**

   Poor gut health is when toxins, undigested food, and harmful bacteria are able to pass through your digestive tract. Collagen gets hard at work to soothe the intestinal lining and immerse it with healing amino acids.

5) **Strengthens your bones**

   We all need and understand the importance of calcium in our diet. Bones are actually made of collagen, so adding this to your diet is beneficial.

Boost Your Health!
Ideas to Add Collagen powder into your day:

» **Smoothies**
» **Melt into your oatmeal**
» **Mix into coffee, tea, or morning elixir**
» **Stir a spoonful into a glass of water**
» **Add-in while baking**

CACAO NIBS –
A CHOCOLATE LOVER'S DELIGHT!

Cacao nibs are a delicious treat with a healthy twist. Cacao is the source for original chocolate production before anything else is added to sweeten the taste. The nibs are cacao beans that have been roasted, separated from their husks, and broken into smaller pieces. They have a deep chocolate flavor that some consider bitter and nutty.

The raw, organic cacao seed is considered a superfood, containing a variety of powerful nutrients, minerals, antioxidants — and, bonus! — zero sugar.

Cacao Nibs Contain:

» Magnesium
» Protein
» Fibre
» Iron
» Sulfur
» Copper
» Zinc
» Potassium
» Antioxidants

Cacao Nib Benefits:

1) **Nutritional powerhouse**
Celebrate chocolate! Raw, organic cacao nibs are an excellent source of iron and fibre. They are also full of protective antioxidants and magnesium.

1) **Food for the brain**

They contain: magnesium for memory; calcium for nerve cell conduction; potassium to help increase thinking ability and concentration; iron in the blood to bring oxygen to the brain; and copper and zinc for brain development. Organic cacao nibs are one smart snack!

2) **Mood enhancer**

Cacao contains compounds that increase endorphins and serotonin levels in the brain. These are the chemicals that cheer you up, reduce anxiety, and give us a sense of well-being.

3) **Natural aphrodisiac**

Think about Valentine's day and boxes of chocolate! The chemicals in the raw bean stimulate the senses and increase feelings of joy and pleasure.

4) **Maintain muscle and nerve function**

Cacao beans are high in magnesium, which is important to muscle and nerve function.

Enjoy Cacao Nibs & Add Them to Anything:

» **Eat raw with nuts**
» **Mix into trail mix**
» **Spoon into oatmeal or cereal**
» **Scatter over ice cream**
» **Drop a pinch onto toast with nut butter**

> You can also grind the cacao nibs and add them to your favorite warm beverage. They don't offer a strong chocolate flavor, but the nutrient punch is worth it.

CACAO BUTTER — STRENGTHEN YOUR SKIN!

Just as cacao nibs are good for us, so is cacao butter — both internally and externally. You have probably seen this ingredient in your skincare but have not realized that you may have eaten it, too! The oil is extracted from the cacao bean and used in the production of chocolate. It has a rich (dark) chocolate kind of flavour with a silky texture.

Cacao butter is known as a healthy fat. Cacao butter is a very "stable" fat, meaning it isn't likely to spoil or become rancid when heated. As a saturated fat, it retains its nutrients and chemical composition easily when used in cooking. This helps to preserve many of the nutritional benefits.

Cacao Butter Contains:

» **Antioxidants**
» **Vitamin K**
» **Vitamin E**

Cacao Butter Benefits:

1) **Prevents dry skin**
   Cacao butter makes an excellent skin moisturizer. To create a more spreadable form, just heat it up in some water, mix with other beneficial products like coconut oil, and apply to your skin. Always do a patch test, just in case.

2) **Heals chapped lips**
   Cacao butter is an emollient, meaning it adds a protective layer of hydration when applied. It is great for the outdoors in cold temperatures and protects against sun damage and any indoor heat that can leave your lips dry and

peeling. I keep a piece on my bedside table for easy application morning and night.

3) **Reduces inflammation**

It offers quick and soothing relief on inflamed skin and has a wonderful aroma.

4) **Mood enhancer**

Cacao contains compounds that increase endorphins and serotonin levels in the brain. These are the chemicals that cheer you up, reduce anxiety, and give us a sense of well-being.

5) **Makes a great shaving cream**

You can use cacao butter in your shower or sink to shave and hydrate your skin at the same time. It melts easily in warm water and won't clog your drain.

Enjoy Cacao Butter & Use it Daily:

» **Use it as an oil; warm it up**
» **Blend it into your hot beverages**
» **Include it in baking**
» **Make your own chocolate**
» **Rub it onto lips for a moisturizing effect**

Cacao butter is great for naturally healing dry, sensitive skin. Slather it onto skin for the entire family.

GREEN SUPERFOOD POWDER — TO THE RESCUE

Green superfood powder has been around since the 1970s. The hippies were on the right track! You can use a juicer and fresh vegetables to make your own green juice, if you have the time. But as a busy mom, working professional, and health conscious woman, I need a different option in my kitchen. So I supplement with beneficial green powder every day. I know that my diet does not contain enough fruit and vegetables no matter how hard I try.

The Green Powders Offer:

1) Nutrient rich superfoods
2) Probiotics
3) Multiple servings of fruit and vegetables
4) Lots of vitamins and minerals
5) A boost of energy and support with natural weight loss

Bottoms UP! Add Green Powder to:

» **Smoothies**
» **Water**
» **Juice (not citrus though)**

My recipe: Fill the blender with coconut water, coconut milk, water, frozen fruit, chia seeds, a scoop of collagen, flax meal, hemp hearts, MCT oil, a scoop of protein powder, and a scoop of green powder. I can't say enough good things about green powder. As silly as it sounds, I notice a difference in my energy levels after finishing a glass. It revives me from the afternoon slump and awakens my weary legs.

FISH OIL — KEEP ON SWIMMING

How much fish do you eat? In my house, we aim for once a week. It is not a favorite meal at our table, so we supplement. I understand the importance of fish in my diet, so I consume fish oil every day.

Fish Oil contains:

» Omega-3EPA - eicosapentaenoic acid
» DHA - docosahexaenoic acid
» Both EPA & DHA are considered essential fatty acids since our bodies can't produce them and they must be acquired through our diets.

Benefits of Fish Oil:

1) Cardiovascular health
2) Brain function & memory
3) Strong bones & teeth
4) Joint health
5) Muscle repair & recovery

May the Fish be With You – Ideas to Add Fish Oil Into Your Day:

» Pour some into your smoothie or protein shake
, » Just take a spoonful
» Grab it in supplement form

The oil comes from the tissues of oily fish. Fish consume Omega-3 oils in their diet of algae and plankton. A spoonful a day works for me. Purchase the lemon flavor; it is light and refreshing with no fishy aftertaste.

MCT OIL — FUEL FOR BRAIN AND BODY

MCT oil stands for medium-chain triglycerides, also known as medium-chain fatty acids, which are widely known as beneficial nutrients for the body. MCTs are a high source of essential healthy fats. The oil is digested easily and travels down to your liver, where it is burned by the body for energy, or "fuel," instead of being stored as fat.

Benefits of MCT Oil:

1) Reduces fatigue
2) Improves energy levels and mood
3) Improves digestion and nutrient absorption
4) Helps protect heart health
5) Improves brain function

Get Clever with MCT — Lots of Ideas For Use:

» **Pour some into your smoothie**
» **Blend into your morning coffee**
» **Whisk together for salad dressing**
» **Take a spoonful anytime**

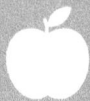

MCT Oil is easy to digest and quickly absorbs into your bloodstream. It is then delivered to your liver where it is converted into energy.

MCT oil is best stored in a cool, dry, dark cupboard. Keep it away from direct sunlight and any heat.

COCONUT OIL — TROPICAL TREE

Coconut oil is a healthy saturated fat; a medium-chain fatty acid. We love coconut oil in my house. I must have a jar in every room. It is so versatile and can be used for natural medicine, cooking, skin care, essential oils, consumption, and so much more.

Benefits of Coconut Oil:

1) Increases energy
2) Boosts the immune system
3) Improves hair and skin health
4) Antibacterial, antifungal, and antiviral properties

Get Tropical with Coconut Oil

In Food:

1) **Cooking at high heat (sautéing and frying)** - Coconut oil is great for cooking at a high heat. Coconut oil is made up of healthy saturated fats so it remains stable under high temperatures.

2) **Coffee or hot beverage** — This is the only way I drink hot beverages anymore! Adding it to your mug not only will give you an energy boost, but the healthy saturated fat will make you feel full longer (but not in a bloated way).

3) **Baking** — Yes, you can bake with coconut oil. Replace the amount of butter or vegetable oil that is called for in the recipe with coconut oil. Also use coconut oil to grease baking sheets, cake pans, or muffin tins, and your delicious baking will simply slide right out.

For Skin:

1) **Moisturizer**

   Coconut oil is fantastic for the skin. I like to apply it after the shower or before bed, but anytime is a great time to lather it on.

2) **Makeup remover**

   Use a small amount of coconut oil on a cotton pad to remove eye makeup.

3) **Wound balm**

   Coconut oil speeds up the healing of rashes, burns, and open wounds. The antibacterial and antifungal properties help to keep the area free of infection. It is great for diaper rash!

For Household:

1) **Removes gum from hair or furniture**
2) **Dust collector & preventer**
3) **Shoe shine**

> Helps the Family Pet – Dogs and cats can benefit from coconut oil added to their diet too. It helps with digestive upset, skin irritations, and wounds. Apply it directly to their skin or add to food. The great thing is that coconut oil is edible, so there is no harm if they lick it off their fur.

As you can see, the benefits of coconut oil are endless. There are so many other uses not listed here. What I love the most is that it is cheap and sold everywhere.

These are just a few of my many nutritious additions that I attempt to incorporate on a daily basis. Every little bit helps!

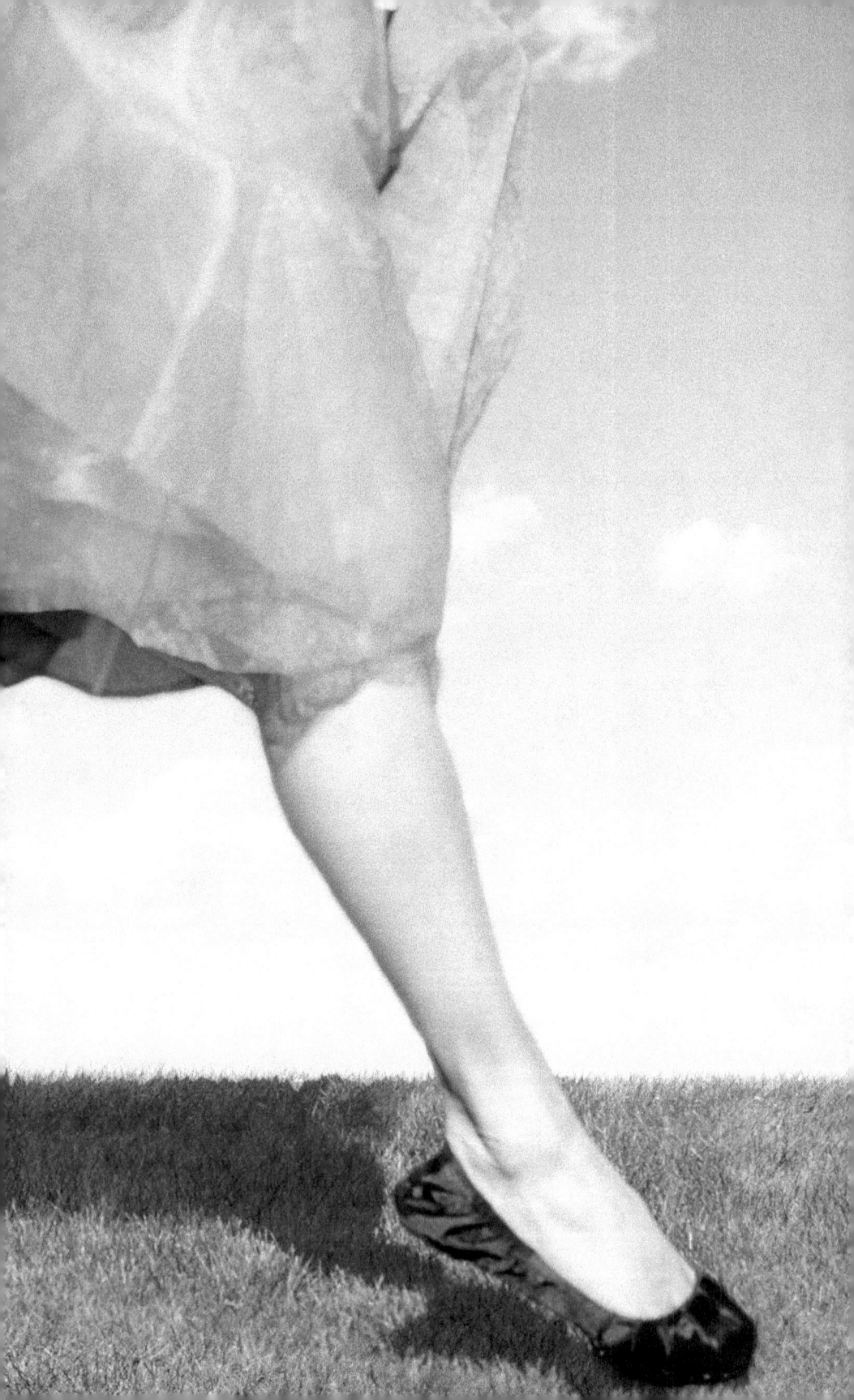

Part Four
GETTING CREATIVE

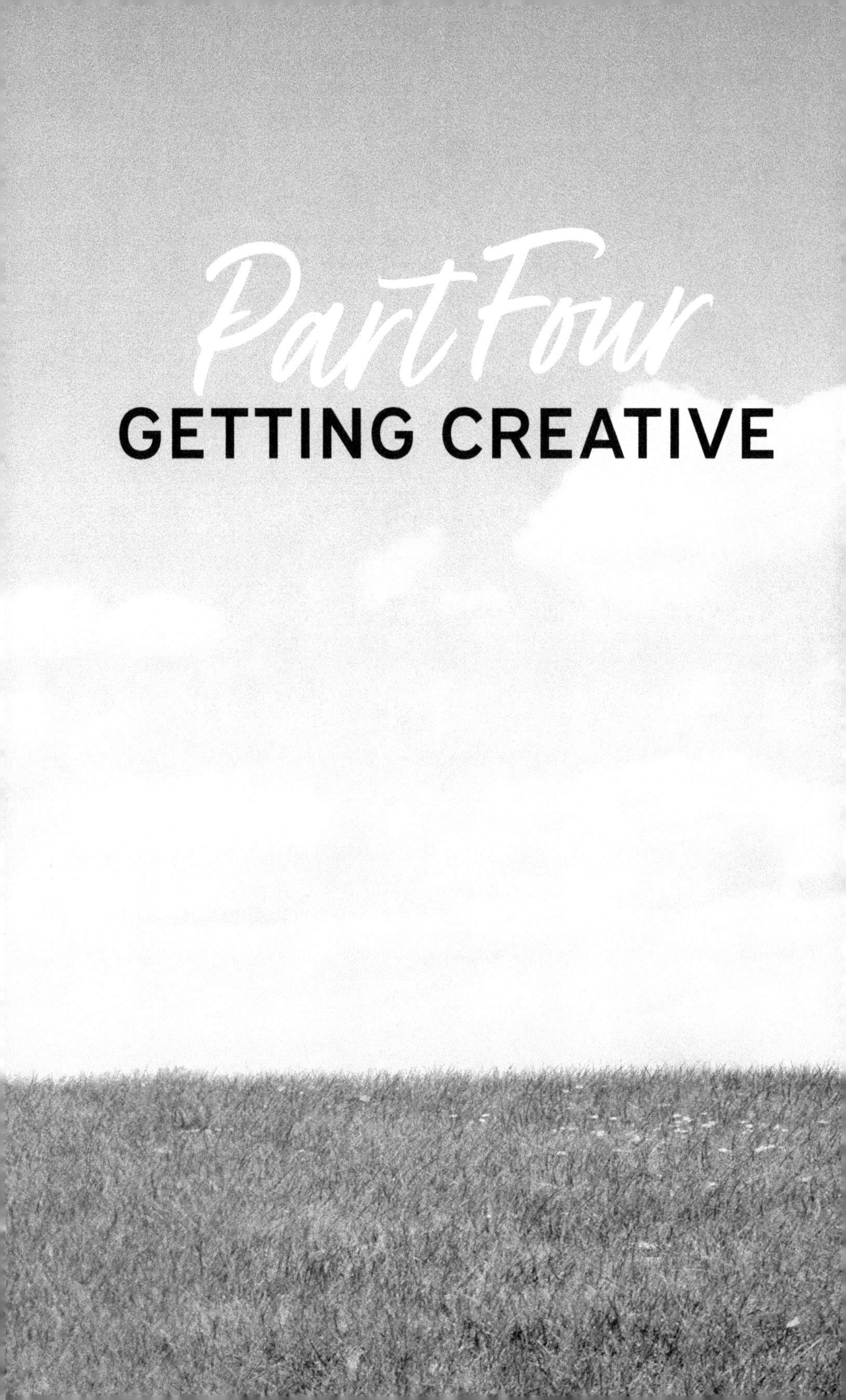

11

Organize, Simplify, Tidy, or Toss!

I love to tidy, put things in piles, move stuff around, de-clutter drawers, buy more than one of something (especially if it is on sale), move plants/flowers around, and get table tops, counters, dressers, and shelves organized. That way I know where things are. God help the human or animal in the house who has moved anything to a secondary location without telling me!

When it comes to organizing, I enjoy the planning process, the creative flair, the charts, the plan, and all of the check-lists that are involved. Actually, I get the biggest thrill out of designing a colourful clip-art-themed template to use. The joy is in the creation process and then printing off the final paper product. I feel prepared to tackle every room and have a plan to follow so I don't get distracted.

It might be due to my health, or probably just the fact that I am getting older, but I crave simplicity in my life. A simple life holds a different meaning for everyone. For me it means elim-inating noise from the outside world, remaining positive in my day-to-day actions, removing items that are creating clutter in my space, and spending time doing what is important to me.

This has the potential to be a big chapter, but hey, I will attempt to keep it simple and give you some ideas, thoughts, or "ahh yes!" moments that you feel make sense. It's a journey that allows you to move forward and a plan that I never stop working on.

YOUR HOME

I believe that you have to let go of the old things to allow room for new things to come into your life. By this I mean possessions that have no real value to you anymore. Maybe they did at one point in your life, but life changes. We grow (literally) and need to create space for updated items. I am not talking about antiques or family heirlooms. As I write this, I look around my office and can locate five things immediately that need to be put out in the recycling box tonight. It is easy to leave them, ignore them, or just forget about them. But this process will change your life! It will open up space in your environment. Lack of space might be dragging you down or even hindering actual physical movement.

Start by working in every room in your house (plan for one room a day, or one a weekend). Go around the room and eliminate anything that is unnecessary. Open all closets and drawers. Be honest with yourself; will you really wear that again? Do you need to keep that article you clipped out of the newspaper anymore? Purge your stuff.

HOME TASKS

Think of all the "make" work tasks you create at home. This list often gets longer than we ever expect. We love to invent work at home. As a mom, wife, and multitasker...I feel the need to stay busy all the time. I tend to feel guilty if I just sit and do nothing.

The home tasks should be shared (in theory). In a household of four, many of the jobs can be delegated or even eliminated once proper consideration is taken. We do not need to do everything ourselves. So start to simplify your home tasks and talk to your family members about what responsibilities will be shared.

YOU ARE IMPORTANT

Learn to evaluate your commitments and time. Look at everything you do in your life. Think of *everything*: making lunches, loading laundry, grocery shopping, working, booking appointments, school activities, sports/dance arrangements, car pool, cooking dinner, cleaning, and keeping a busy family running smoothly. Moms are often overworked and underpaid. Now think about which activities you *value*. What do you *love* doing?

Measure your time. How are you spending most of your waking hours? What are you wasting time on? What can you eliminate from your daily to-do list that weighs your spirit down? Now think of all of the wonderful habits that you can add to your day that would align with your soul and give you purpose.

Here is a hard one, but a crucial tactic for self-preservation: learn to say NO. You have to come first, so put yourself there and say no to the many distractions, requests, and demands that are put upon you. Love yourself enough to make YOU a priority in your day.

REGULATE THE TECHNOLOGY

In the 21st century, electronics have taken over — mostly in amazing ways, though. Technology offers so many benefits, but it can be overwhelming when trying to reduce stimulation and attempting to create more contentment in our lives.

Keep your email inbox clean. All of the advertising emails, the sale alerts, and notifications are not necessary. Hit "unsubscribe" for messages that have no importance. Once you read a message, delete it or save it to a file for the future. This way you lift a weight off of your shoulders, as you no longer have to think about your messages piling up.

Control your communications and set up boundaries to protect yourself. Just because you have a cell phone, Twitter, Facebook, or Instagram account does not mean that you have to be available 24/7. Unless it is an emergency, you can get back to someone after you arrive at your destination, when your exercise program is done, or once you've finished your lunch. (I am talking about your personal life communications and web surfing, not your work responsibilies.)

I tend to enjoy games on my phone. I can easily talk myself into thinking that they are helping me work my brain. They are, but breaks are necessary as I need to get up and move.

Give yourself some time away from your phone, if you can. Sundays work for me. Concentrate on the family, do things you enjoy, and recharge for the new week that is fast approaching.

SLOW DOWN AND FORGET THE SMALL STUFF

Despite all of your efforts — whether you have an illness, a busy family, or a thriving career — you cannot be in constant motion. You need to know when to rest and take some precious time for yourself. This is not being lazy; this is being proactive for you! Did you hear that? FOR YOU. Learn to identify what really matters in your day, what has meaning, and what doesn't.

OWN LESS AND BE FRUGAL

Everyone likes a good deal (I love sales). With email alerts, and the convenience of Amazon, it is easy to get caught up in the online shopping frenzy. Technology is fantastic, but it is so simple to get carried away and fill up your cart. You don't want to miss that promotion; it ends in 24 hours! But how much do you really need? How much can your pantry actually store? Make sure that anything you have in your life has a reason to be there and offers something in return. The more junk you own, the more it starts to take over.

EAT WELL AND MOVE

Without proper nutrition, your body will not function at its best. Try (yes, make an effort) to eat well throughout the day and find the time to exercise. Don't make this hard and say that you don't have the time. Consume some protein for breakfast, enjoy three pieces of fruit a day, and a handful of veggies for lunch and dinner. Then pick a movement for 30 minutes, if you can, to get some exercise. Go for a walk (inside or outside). Do some stretches. Lift some weights. Use the stairs or dance. Eating well and exercising will help build a healthy body and mind.

CREATE A MEAL PLAN

If figuring out your family's daily meals is a stressor for you as you manage cooking time around school, work, sports, and transportation, then create a weekly menu plan. Choose simple lunches and dinners, go grocery shopping, and record the menu on a calendar. Now you have weekly meals planned out, ingredients purchased, and preparation times scheduled. (See page 101 for more on this!)

SELF-EXPRESSION AND INNER SIMPLICITY

Let the fun begin. Learn to spend some time alone and re-charge. Solitude is a blessing. Enjoy the quiet time to reflect, gain focus, and renew your spirit. You can use this time to meditate, journal, sit outside, or listen to music.

Create a space in a room — on a bedside table or in a quiet corner — that is your special place. We moved a chair into the corner of our dining room because it gets the morning sun. Then I get to enjoy the sunshine for ten minutes to get ready for the day.

Surround it with visuals that uplift you, fresh flowers, motivational quotes, and scents that empower you. Vision boards are great to use. Find a creative outlet for self-expression. Draw, paint, color, write, dance, or design on the computer — whatever it is, it will lift your mood and can even reduce stress.

DESIGN MORNING & EVENING ROUTINES

Follow a daily routine that helps to simplify your time. This can be a quick reflection in the morning, daily mantras, recording thoughts in a journal at night, or stretching before you climb into bed. Fill your time with simple pleasures that generate peace in your day.

§

It sounds so simple, right? Adopt your own version of a simpler life. Concentrate on what you need to be healthy, and spread love. These are some items that work for me, but the options are endless. Start small and enjoy the journey.

SNOW DAY

*L*et's talk about the weather. Never before has the weather played such a deciding factor in my daily life. Okay, that's a lie. Who am I kidding? The weather has always affected my fashion, hair style, and footwear choices.

Too hot and humid — Ponytail to deal with the frizz and curls and strappy sandals. ***Raining and wet*** — Baseball hat to keep hair dry and ankle boots or cute rain boots. ***Snowing*** — Stylish winter hat and luxurious winter boots with fur cuffs.

Aww, those were the days! Now all of my choices and any plans for the day have to include my safety. The last thing my family or I want is for me to fall and hurt myself. I have to consider every aspect of leaving the house: literally the clothes I put on, the path to my car, the entrance at the potential location, any inside and outside mobility issues, and the projected weather forecast.

Because it snowed today, I am focused on that issue. I actually dread snow, which makes me feel guilty as my kids dream of snow days and no school! Don't get me wrong, I love the look of snow. The peaceful picture it paints when collected on the tree tops. The thought of a cozy fireplace warming up the house. As I look out the window today, all I see is an obstacle and I wonder if I have the energy to overcome the path ahead of me.

My family is fantastic, as they ensure that my car and the walkway is cleared of snow and ice before they leave for work or school. I am truly grateful for how they protect me. It is not always the prospect of leaving my house that stresses me out, though. It is the aspects still unknown about my arrival location. I have to be prepared for anything. The whole thought process can be daunting sometimes.

Here is where my life has changed over the last 25 years —
and snow is an aggressive reminder. Most days I use a cane
outside of the house and I expect it to balance me on any
surface. Ice is another sneaky story. Will the cane slide out
from under me? Will I slip and fall? Has the store cleared the
snow and ice from the door? Will I just stay in the car and drive
back home? Trust me, I have done that, folks.

Until you have a mobility issue, snow days are never a concern
— just an annoyance, really. Brush the snow off the car, shovel
the driveway, traffic issues, snow tires, windshield wipers,
antifreeze, and defrost. I still have to deal with all of that, in
addition to having to decide if I am leaving the house at all. Is
there an emergency to deal with? Do we need groceries that
bad? Can I work from home?

I often get asked if a certain season is harder on my MS. Well,
that depends. If the summer is too hot and humid, it slows
me right down and drains all of the energy from my core. So
I tend to stay inside, out of the sun and in the safety of air
conditioning. If the winter is too messy, it also keeps me inside,
out of the snow and enjoying the fireplace. Wow, I am inside a
lot! I prefer the spring and fall seasons, obviously. My energy is
up and I can get out of the house more often.

All year long obstacles surround me. I have to learn ways to
deal with them and move (literally) forward. My daily plans have
to work around the weather. Creating my to-do list is fun, but
it has to be adaptable to what is outside my window. Doctor's
appointments or grocery shopping often get swapped with
baking and laundry if Mother Nature is not cooperating. But
that's okay because it is my decision to do what is right for me!

12

Daily Affirmations

*H*ave you ever practiced a daily affirmation exercise? I practice, repeat, and write them down every day. Affirmations have the power to guide you, help you to concentrate on achieving your goals, give you the power to change your negative thinking patterns (which is daily with an autoimmune illness), and replace them with positive thoughts. By saying affirmations out loud (or in your head), in front of a mirror, or writing them down, you affirm your thoughts and direct your brain to respond in a positive way.

If the idea that you can change the way you think about yourself by repeating some positive phrases might feel a little foolish, I get it. I totally get it. How will words make my health improve? Generally speaking, they won't. I realized it wasn't going to cure anything, but instead would help change how I think of myself and the effect that my illness has over me.

To understand how affirmations work, it helps to first know some of the science behind how we think. Yes, this is a science. The human brain is made of billions of neurons, which are cells that send messages between the different brain regions, all with various functions to perform. Your brain is a very busy organ.

When you think, neurons fire electrical impulses along pathways in your brain, which makes those neurons more sensitive and strengthens the pathways. In contrast, the brain will eventually trim the connections between neurons when those pathways aren't used enough. So let's build strong pathways by repeatedly thinking about something positive, making it easier to fall into that thought process in the future.

Your thoughts influence your actions on a daily basis. What you think about, you bring about. For example, the more you affirm to yourself that you are confident, the more you will begin to stop thinking that you can't do something and realize you are capable of completing tasks that were once difficult. It is a belief in yourself.

Choose phrases that are meaningful to you, repeat them, and take action based on your affirmations. Create an affirmation practice. Set aside time in the morning and evening to complete the process. Affirmations can be a powerful and life changing tool. Over time, what you repeatedly tell yourself does have the ability to shape how you think and feel.

The important thing is to find affirmations that resonate with you. I personally like starting all of mine with the words "I AM" or "I HAVE." Usually I like to begin and end my day reciting them to myself. I also use this tool anytime I feel stressed, anxious, sad, or angry.

I AM HEALTHY
I take care of my body and mind with food, exercise, nature, and rest.

I AM ALIVE
I am living an extraordinary life full of love, peace, and joy.

I AM PROUD

I have raised two incredible, vibrant, respectful, & healthy kids.

I AM POWERFUL

I have the courage to live a life I love.

I HAVE THRIVED

I did not let MS stop me.

When you practice them daily, repeat them, write them out, and believe in them, you will start to see changes in your everyday mindset. Thanks to affirmations, I am able to sit in the dentist's chair, with periodic breaks, but I am still able to get my teeth cleaned!

13

Create a Vision Board

I love this visionary project. It is fun, creative, and really easy to do. How you envision yourself, your day, and your life is so important. What you tell yourself you will believe, so why not put some motivational thoughts in that brain of yours and create the best life you can?

Everyone in your house can do this. I use it to motivate myself each day and my kids even create one for their yearly goals. We hang them in places where we will see them each day as a constant reminder for us to get inspired.

A vision board is an incredible visualization tool. It is a very powerful snapshot of your vision of the future. What are your dreams, your hopes, or your goals for your life? You can create one each year to help guide you on your path and then celebrate the visions that came to life.

NOW THE FUN BEGINS: CREATING YOUR VISION BOARD

Start by researching other vision boards if you need some ideas or inspiration. The internet is a wealth of examples. I have more than one board in my house: one to motivate me personally, a professional board that includes career goals, my kids use them for school or sports accomplishments, and I have another for nutrition and exercise goals to visualize the physical changes I am working towards. There are so many others I want to create. It becomes an addiction of inspiration.

Start by finding pictures that express the feelings, possessions, or events that you want to attract into your life. You can create them on the computer, a Bristol board, a binder, or a regular sheet of paper. Use whatever you have handy. This process is so much fun! It is like scrapbooking, except you are creating a future, not reliving one.

Find pictures in magazines, photographs, photos from the internet, and even ones your kids have drawn. It needs to inspire you and encourage you to stay focused on positive thoughts. Illness and the various daily struggles can bring you down, so you need to find a way to lift yourself up.

Consider including family pictures or even photos of yourself. Do you have a pet? Photos of you laughing? The kids being silly? The goal is to use anything that makes you feel good and that brings a smile to your face. What you place on your board and think about each day will be attracted to you. So plan it out, spend some time on it, and have fun.

I also like to include motivational quotes, inspirational words, or sayings that move me. Sometimes it is lyrics from a favorite song, sayings from a favorite movie, jokes, or a person that I look up to. Be creative; add color, designs, graphics, shapes, and lines. This is your work of art.

Keep it simple. Don't clutter too much on the board. I like it to be neat. Each picture has a border around it and they are all square shaped. They can be overlapping, on angles, or used as a border. I like it to look symmetrical and balanced.

HOW TO USE YOUR VISION BOARD

Where you put your boards is very important. Now that you have spent so much energy on this project, you want to be able to see it every day. Put them in locations that you will be in regularly. I have my main life vision board on the fridge, so every time I am in the kitchen, I can see it, read it, experience the emotions it provokes, and attract those dreams to my consciousness. Then I have one in my office beside my desk for my business goals. I even have my nutritional and dream boards set up in a binder, which I read through each morning.

I like to start out my day every morning, before the whole family is up, visualizing and focusing on my fridge board. That way it is quiet, the sun is starting to come up, and I can spend time concentrating. Once I get to my office, as the computer is loading, I concentrate on my career board and visualize my goals.

Each year I create new boards, as my goals have changed or many of the goals I had placed on the boards manifested!

An example of one photo on my board was a dolphin leaping out of the water. It is a beautiful picture and one that I enjoyed looking at each day. Months later, we took a family vacation to Cuba and we had the opportunity to swim with dolphins. Moving in the water with these magnificent creatures is an once-in-a-lifetime experience, and I was not passing it up. Those moments change your life. My vision came to life.

I love to reflect back on the boards as well. Doing this allows me to see how much I have grown and accomplished over the years, as my goals from age 25 to 50 have been changed personally and professionally. It reminds me of how far I have come.

MY FINAL REFLECTIONS
ON USING A VISION BOARD

Set aside time each day to gaze at your vision board. Look over every detail and concentrate on what it all represents to you. Say the quotes and motivational words out loud, if you can. Visualize acquiring or experiencing all that you have placed on it. Believe that what you have designed will come to you. Most of all, be grateful and say thank you to the universe for all of the gifts that you currently have.

TO PARK OR
NOT TO PARK?

This is a difficult topic. Yes, I have Multiple Sclerosis, but I am not handicapped! I am sure you are similar to me and were taught to respect other people, so I would never consider parking in an accessible parking spot. I have two legs and can walk perfectly fine with a cane (as I stumble and veer to the right with each step). Hell, I am the person who offers to help any and everyone, if I see them trying to load groceries into their car, pick items off the top shelves, or give them my seat if all others are taken. So, no, I am not handicapped. I am a lucky one who gets to walk around freely each day (but check with me tomorrow and my legs might have a different plan for me).

I remember trying to justify applying for an accessible parking permit. I am a planner, so I actually did this prior to needing the use of a cane. According to the government website, you must qualify according to various health conditions. Multiple Sclerosis falls under the neurological category with severely limited mobility. Okay... but I am not severely limited, so would any doctor even certify that my health condition qualifies for this permit? I have the MRI scans to prove that I suffer from this disabling disease, but just by looking at me, no one would have any idea.

How could I walk (keyword: walk) into the government office and hand in the paperwork to apply for such a permit? Isn't the teller going to look me up and down? Sizing me up, thinking I am a fraud or a fake? Talk about me on her lunch break? Get annoyed with healthy people like me who abuse the system? Okay, I am overthinking this scenario way too much. The teller probably couldn't care less, and she is just waiting for her lunch break to come. I am being polite and trying to crack a joke or two while she enters the information into the computer and hands me the temporary permit to place on my windshield. Then she calls "next!" and I walk out of the office, not being noticed by anyone. But I still turn around to see if anyone is watching me carrying the permit in my right hand.

So life begins with a handicapped permit. It is interesting how this plays out in my head. I don't need this. Okay, sometimes I do, but not all the time. So am I a part-time handicapped person? I'm not fully committed to the definition it represents. I have been called many things in my life: daughter, sister, dancer, teacher, realtor, wife, mother...but never handicapped. I don't want to be labeled as this. I don't want anyone to feel sorry for me and my life journey. I don't want people to treat me differently or think that there is anything I cannot do. So I put the permit into the glove compartment and vow to only use it when I am at my worst.

I think back on my healthy, active lifestyle. How could I be needing to park in handicapped parking? This is all part of my battle with my body over how it is going to change or be affected. So much of how I live is in contradiction to my diagnosis back in 1996.

It took me a few weeks before I could gather up the courage (nerve, you might say) to park in said designated location at the mall. Upon arriving, my legs are feeling good, but stiff from the drive (as that seems to happen now once I have been sitting for any length of time — it takes about 15 minutes really).

I park, check all of the windows, make sure no one is around, slowly get out of the car, and make my way to the entrance doors. Should I walk fast to get there before anyone witnesses this parking crime that I have committed? Or just realize that no one is around or watching me, so just walk inside? My thoughts and heart are racing until I feel the rush of air conditioning greeting me inside. Only then can I relax. My trips to the mall were limited as it was, so this scenario didn't play out very much.

Fast-forward to my current life, and as my usual days go, I am mobile unless I have done too much. And going to a store can be thought of as too much. I tend to have my route. I know what locations work best for me. Parking is available right by the door, and I know where the bathrooms are once I'm inside. It takes a while for the shopping to be completed, and then I am on my way out. By this time my legs are tired, my left leg begins to drag, the cane is leaned on more, and quite often I stumble, trip, or wobble.

I see my car! Ta-da! The light at the end of the tunnel. Only a few more steps and I am in the safety of my vehicle. Now if there is a curb of any kind, I have to concentrate on my footing so I don't fall. Upon closing the car door, I turn on the engine, adjust the volume on the radio, and say a small "thank you" for letting the store experience be a good one (and over). It is then that I realized that maybe parking in this spot is what I needed after all– even if I still looked around to see if anyone was watching me.

Conclusion

*A*fter working hard for years to create this personal/infor-
mative/helpful yet entertaining book, my life took over.
Life, in every sense of the word: my Real Estate career, my
health, my kids growing up and one graduating high school,
my parents, our dog, the house, our cars, the groceries, the
cooking, the bills, the pandemic, the list goes on and on. You
get it, because you live it, too.

It was time to concentrate on myself and my environment because I felt like it was spinning out of control (weird, as I
was writing a book about myself this whole time). It probably
wasn't, but from my point of view, it was. My mind doesn't
work the same way. I tend to get overwhelmed, exhausted,
annoyed, angry, frustrated and emotional much quicker than I
used to.

I started reading stuff on MS and how I am supposed to be
feeling. So yeah, I am exhausted (just like that blog said), and
I am bloated (just like that podcast on menopause mentioned),
and I don't sleep well (again, just like that book focused on).
WAIT! As you can see, I got lost in all the media conversations
taking place on a daily basis: the Instagram posts, the Tweets,
the Facebook posts, the Google news stories, the bestselling
books, etc.

If you are like me, I blame everything on my illness.

Sore hip? MS — *really my sleep position.*

Headache? MS — *actually the weather system*

Exhausted? MS — *honestly just me, as I keep too busy*

Terrible sleep? MS — *actually my cute little dog, who takes up too much room on the bed and keeps me awake*

Angry? MS — *probably just overwhelmed, then angry with myself for being angry*

Trust me, when I was first diagnosed, I purchased, borrowed, and researched anything and everything about this mystery illness that I knew nothing about (there was no social media back then). All I envisioned was a wheelchair. It was hard to absorb the information and not compare myself to others. As we all know, no two illnesses are ever the same. The medical world will label it the same way, but my experiences of a flare-up might be nothing like yours. And the lasting effects, if any, are incredibly different.

I have decided that I am done — and I am letting go of all that industry hype around Multiple Sclerosis health. Personally, I don't have enough time to listen, read, attend, follow, or chat with all the information outlets that are designed to help me. I needed to get back to ME and what has worked for ME in the past by living the life that supports ME.

I needed to take a break and try to deal with all of the new challenges that have come my way. After thriving for over 20 years with an illness that consumed my every thought, I started to experience sustained weakness in my left leg. It was becoming a challenge to walk without holding onto the walls, chairs, counters, stairs, or people around me.

So the emotional shopping for a cane began (and when I say "emotional" — I mean it). It took more than one trip to even enter the store. It was hard to get over that hurdle of acceptance for needing a device to hold me up. (I used to dance in Character Shoes, people. Those have heels!) I didn't want to look weak or as though I needed help. I can do it; watch me!

Then within a few more years, I began to use an ankle brace for my drop foot and a scooter was added to my transportation devices so that I could join my family on daily walks around the neighbourhood. And again, wow! My struggle to even sit on this new form of transportation was heartbreaking for me to admit. I know it is only a scooter, and I am still so grateful that I only needed to introduce this mobility equipment now. But I felt like a failure, as though everything I had done to sustain my health failed. I know it hasn't. Every step forward in my illness matters for my future. These tools help keep me safe and active every day.

You may or may not align with the choices I've made. But we all have to do what is right for us, what we truly believe is the best option for our own health. I started my journey on a drug and found it did not work for me. Luckily, I have built up a fantastic support team that I draw knowledge from on a regular basis. I trust their advice and follow any directions shared with me in my everyday life. I have bravely lived half of my life while exploring and controlling my symptoms with their guidance.

Writing this book genuinely kept me healthy, focused, upbeat, and energetic each day. I am writing a book — it's a dream come true. My plan was to share all of the strategies, tips, and approaches that I have included into my life over the years (plus people kept telling me that I am an inspiration). I hope something in this book inspires you, awakens your warrior spirit, or provides you with the encouragement necessary to move forward on your own journey.

Thank you for reading my book, and good luck on your path.

References

Axe, Josh MD. "Health, Wellness and Nutrition." Dr. Axe, 18
   Apr. 2023, draxe.com/.

"DoTERRA Essential Oils." DoTERRA, 1 Jan. 2023,
   doterra.com/CA/en/about-our-story.

Hawley, Gretchen MD. "The MSing Link with Dr. Gretchen
   Hawley." The MSing Link, 18 Apr. 2023,
   doctorgretchenhawley.com/.

Homeopathy 360, homeopathy360.com/. Accessed 6 Jul. 2022.

"Homeopathic Remedies." The Centre for Homeopathic
   Education, 18 Apr. 2023, chehomeopathy.com/blog/.

Martin, Piper. "The Homeopathic Midwife." Piper Martin,
   pipermartin.com/. Accessed 6 Jul. 2022.

Moore, Catherine MBA. "Positive Daily Affirmations: Is There
   Science Behind It?" Positive Psychology, 4 Mar. 2019,
   positivepsychology.com/daily-affirmations/. Accessed 6 Jul.
   2022.

"Our Holistic Herb Approach." St. Francis Herb Farm, 1 Jan. 2023,
   stfrancisherbfarm.com/our-approach/.

Rountree, Robert, et al. Smart Medicine For a Healthier Child:
   The Practical A-to-Z Reference to Natural and Conventional
   Treatments for Infants & Children. 2nd ed., Avery, 2003.

About the Author

Kelli Gastis is an Author and Multiple Sclerosis warrioress. She has been a real estate agent, a dance teacher, a marketing & promotions specialist, a model, a daycare provider, and a fitness enthusiast.

Kelli is a proud mom, wife, sister, and daughter, and loves spending time with family. She enjoys cottages, sitting by the lake, flowers, the spring and fall seasons, reading, collecting daily planners that she saves for no reason, photography, decorating anything, essential oils, and Candy Crush. (She may or may not spend too much time playing that game!)

visit

KelliGastis.com

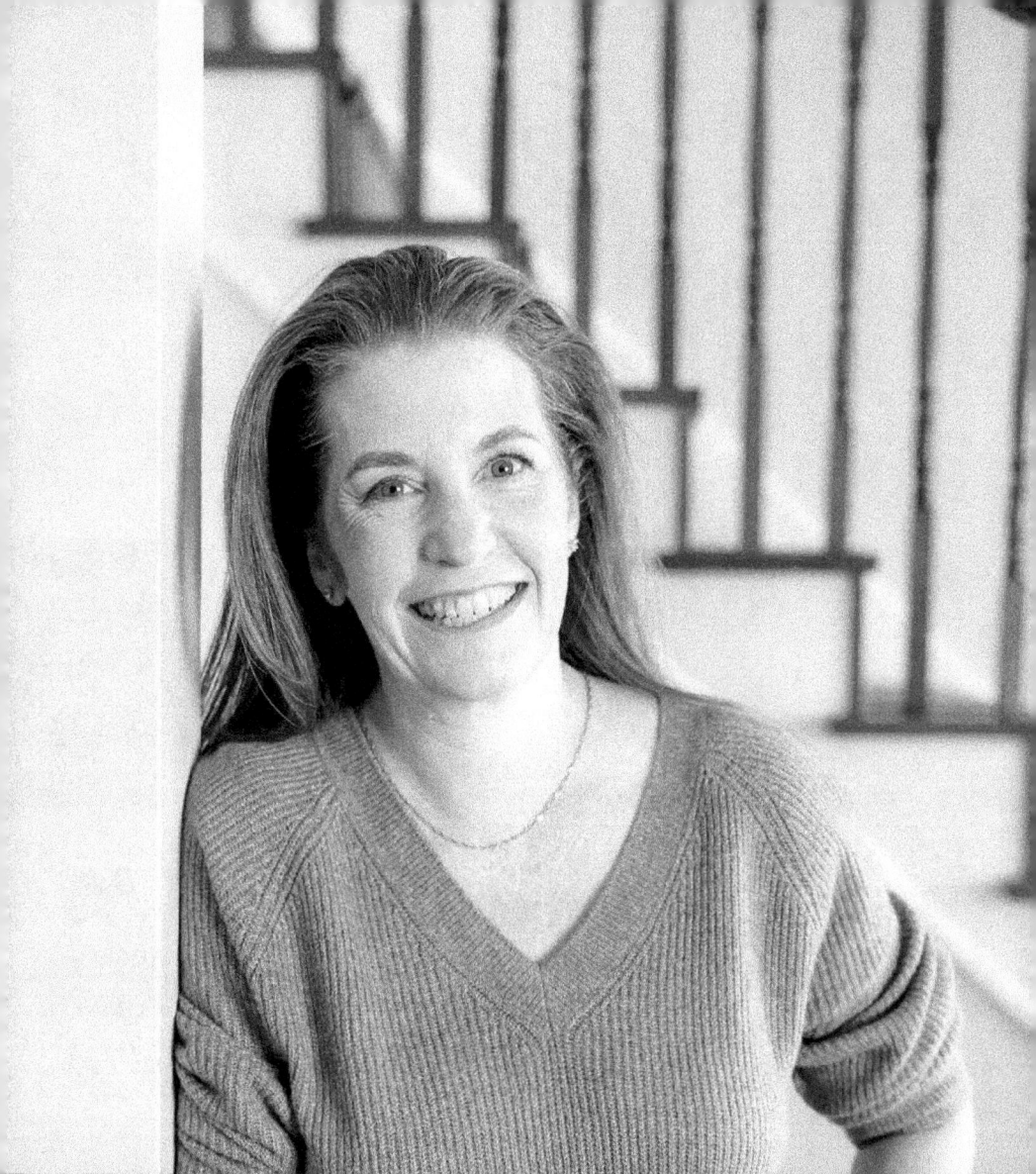

 @KELLIGASTIS

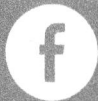 @KELLI.GASTIS

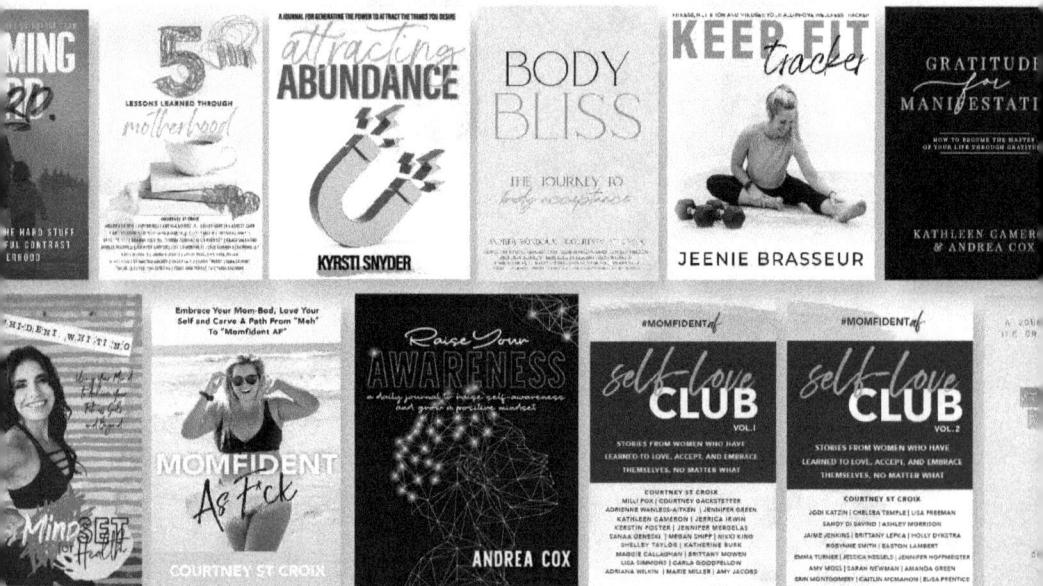